The
Black Parents'
Handbook

Clara J. McLaughlin

With

Donald R. Frisby, M.D.

Richard A. McLaughlin, M.D.

Melvin W. Williams, M.D., M.P.H.

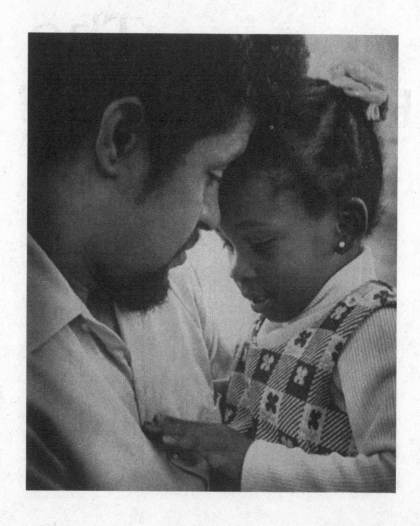

The Black Parents' Handbook

A Guide to Healthy Pregnancy, Birth, and Child Care

A Harvest/HBJ Book
Harcourt Brace Jovanovich, Publishers
San Diego   New York   London

Printed in the United States of America

Picture Credits: Page ii, Virtle S. Bennett; xx, 13, 15, 18, 21, 48, 51, 53, 70,
83, 95, 114, 118, 134, 146, 148, 149, 150, 184, 189, 199, 201, 207, 209,
Jeff Fearing; 5, Nadia Page; 6, reproduced from *Health: Man in a Changing
Environment,* Second Edition, by Benjamin A. Kogan, copyright © 1970, 1974
by Harcourt Brace Jovanovich, Inc.; 28, 31, 90, 112, 139, 154, 156, 164, Kenton
Barnett; 96, 105, 110, Hugh Bell; 120, Dr. Curtis Dilworth; 141, courtesy
of Mrs. Arnetta Jackson; 190, © 1973 by Guidance Associates; 202, Fleming
Mathews III.

Library of Congress Cataloging in Publication Data

McLaughlin, Clara J
 The Black parents' handbook.

 Includes index.
  1. Infants—Care and hygiene. 2. Negro children. 3. Pregnancy.
I. Title. [DNLM: 1. Pregnancy—Popular works. 2. Child Care—Popular works.
WQ150 M161b]
RJ61.M328 649'.1'0242 75-43986
ISBN 0-15-113185-6
  0-15-613100-5 (pbk.)

CDEFGHIJ

To Rinetta, who helped to make the need visible.
And to all black children, hoping that this book
will make their lives more bountiful.

Contents

Part Two

Infant and Child Care

Introduction

Why a book on black child care?

Shortly after I became a mother, I realized that I was not able to use the developmental scales outlined in any of the books on infant care without reading far in advance of my baby's age. I discovered that other black mothers had the same experience. Surveys later conducted by the authors revealed that the average black infant develops mentally and physically at a faster rate than that indicated by the standard infant development scales. The growth patterns described in this book are based on our findings.

Investigation also showed that genetic, medical, and environmental problems common among blacks were not mentioned in books on infant care or even in many medical textbooks. All races suffer from genetic diseases. Among blacks, two of the most serious are sickle cell anemia and hypertension. Umbilical hernias are more frequently found in black infants. So is lead poisoning, an environmental problem. On the other hand, there are illnesses blacks rarely have to face—for example, brain tumors and skin cancer. We have identified the principal health problems encountered by the black community, as well as the problems associated with pregnancy, infancy, and childhood regardless of color.

No book to guide black parents can ignore superstitions and black folk medicine practices. We have included such a section in this book. Our object is to point out practices that could be harmful to the mother and child physically or mentally.

Further, a guide for black parents cannot be truly helpful without dealing with the political and economic influences that affect child rearing. We have considered these issues, too.

The myth of black inferiority is sustained not only by the majority population in the United States, but also by people the world over, who seem to equate blackness with academic, moral, and general incompetence. This myth unquestionably affects the black child mentally.

Many blacks hate themselves for being black. The hate stems from the teachings of this society and is reinforced by economic deprivation, political subjugation, and cultural degradation. Our best teachers of self-hate, however, have often been our own families and friends as they subconsciously disparage blackness.

This book is designed to guide black parents in rearing their children to develop self-esteem and reach their full potential. The roles of both mother and father are important in this mission. The educational and financial status of parents does not affect the early development of the infant, our studies indicate. And it has been proved that children who continue to receive emotional warmth after the first two years of life, regardless of family status, attain greater academic advancement, usually have a higher opinion of themselves, and show a higher regard for others.

If you do not help to motivate your child, he may develop a poor system of values and show little self-respect. For example, if you refuse to answer or ignore questions asked by your child, his innate curiosity and desire to learn will be discouraged. This may eventually lead to a poor performance academically, once he begins school.

Children learn from their environment. Although their parents play the largest part, friends, teachers, and other people with whom they come in contact also influence their lives.

We want you to enjoy becoming parents. Therefore, we have written a complete, easy-to-follow guide, designed to serve your needs from the time your child is conceived until he is six years old.

All of the incidents in this book are real. Only the names have been changed. Many of them may appear negative to readers, but our object is to alert parents to destructive attitudes and practices.

We, the authors, and you, the parents, have the same goal: to save the children. So, read on!

CLARA J. McLAUGHLIN

Acknowledgments

There are so many people to thank for the inspiration and completion of this book that to list them all would mean another publication. Thanks must go, however, to the many black parents who allowed their children to participate in our developmental survey or who consented to have their children photographed. I must also thank the many beautiful black mothers and fathers who read or listened to parts or all of the manuscript.

Very special thanks must go to Dr. Hildrus Poindexter, who spent many hours reading the manuscript during its rough stages as well as writing three of the chapters. Mrs. Marjorie Hooper, teacher and black mother, must also be given many thanks for her research and editorial help.

I am also grateful to my friends who have been understanding and cooperative in so many ways. These include William Gordon, Harold Holmes, Robby Reid, Angela Winfield, Linda Wesley, Carol Mathews, Marilyann Williams, Carmen Francis, Jeneene Kean, and Janice Matthews—the last, not only for her excellent typing skills but also for her dedication.

Sincere thanks must be given to Dave and Arnetta Jackson for their constructive guidance from birth.

Collaborators

Donald R. Frisby, M.D.
Pediatric Dermatologist
Howard University Hospital
Washington, D.C.

Richard A. McLaughlin, M.D.
Obstetrician and Gynecologist
Memorial Hospital System
Houston, Texas

Melvin W. Williams, M.D., M.P.H.
Psychiatrist
National Institute of Mental Health
Rockville, Maryland,
Psychiatric Department
Howard University
Washington, D.C.

Consultants

Robyn J. Arrington, M.D.
Former Member, Board of Trustees, Meharry Medical College
Nashville, Tennessee

John F. J. Clark, M.D.
Chairman, Department of Obsterics and Gynecology
Howard University
Washington, D.C.

W. Montague Cobb, M.D., Ph.D.
Editor, *Journal of the National Medical Association*
Distinguished Professor of Anatomy Emeritus
Howard University
Washington, D.C.

Daniel A. Collins, D.D.S., M.S.D., F.I.C.D.
Oral Pathologist
Consultant to the Surgeon General
San Francisco, California

Curtis Dilworth, D.D.S.
Atlanta, Georgia

Augustus O. Godette, M.D.
Associate Professor of Obstetrics and Gynecology
Howard University,
Medical Officer in Obsterics and Gynecology
D.C. General Hospital
Washington, D.C.

Charles B. Hutchinson, M.D.
Ophthalmologist and Medical Officer
Howard University Hospital
Washington, D.C.

Melvin Jenkins, M.D.
Chairman, Department of Pediatrics and Child Health
Howard University
Washington, D.C.

Fleming Mathews III, M.A.
Social Anthropologist
Washington, D.C.

Harold R. Minus, M.D.
Instructor, Department of Dermatology
Howard University
Washington, D.C.

Hildrus Poindexter, M.D., Ph.D.
Professor of Community Health Practice
Howard University,
Medical Director (Retired) U.S. Public Health Service
Tropical, Medical, and Public Health Specialist
Washington, D.C.

Edward Saunders, M.D.
Urologist
Former Associate Professor of Urology
Howard University,
Consultant to St. Elizabeth Hospital
Washington, D.C.

Jeanne Spurlock, M.D.
Child Psychiatrist
Former Chairman of Psychiatry Department
Meharry Medical College
Nashville, Tennessee,
Deputy Medical Director
American Psychiatric Association
Washington, D.C.

The
Black Parents'
Handbook

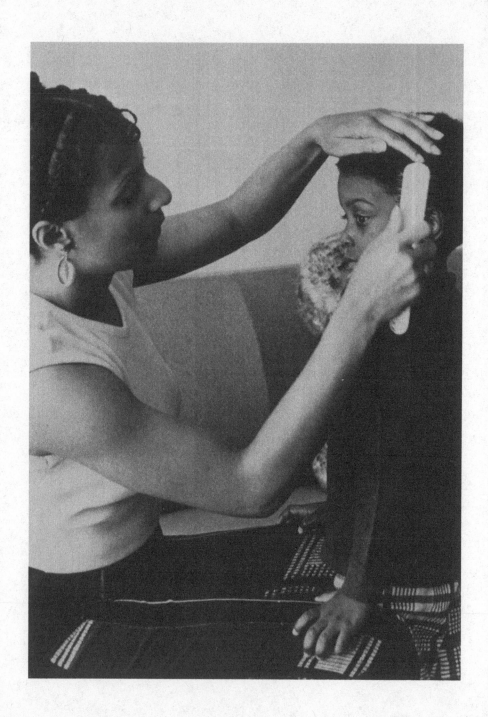

Part One

Black Parents

1

Conception

Alice, a twenty-six-year-old mother of three, had just missed her second period. She suspected another baby was on the way, but could not understand why. Alice told her doctor, "I just can't understand how I got pregnant. I was only with him once without protection, and I didn't even come."

A nurse from a birth-control clinic saw one of her patients whom she had lectured and to whom she had given birth-control pills. She asked the patient if she was still taking the pills. The patient replied, "No, nurse, I don't take them anymore, because my boyfriend takes them for me."

These incidents may appear isolated or unreal. However, they are not. There are many people who understand neither the menstrual cycle nor conception.

Look at yourself for a moment. Can you imagine that you started from a single unfertilized egg about $\frac{1}{200}$ of an inch in diameter plus one sperm even smaller than that little egg? The act of conception is difficult for most of us to imagine, but before we talk about "the making of a baby" let's examine some basic things which precede conception. It is worthwhile to bear in mind that men and women are *complementary*, each supplying what the other needs, each "doing his own thing."

A step-by-step description of the sexual mechanism in the female as well as the male will clarify the complementary role each plays in conception.

The average black female begins to have vaginal bleeding (menstrual flow, or period) about age twelve. Some begin a year or two sooner or a year or two later. At the onset, the cycle may not be regular. In fact, it takes about one year to have regular periods. The menstrual flow usually lasts from 3 to 7 days. The menstrual cycle begins with the first day of bleeding and continues until the onset of the next flow, ranging from 26 to 34 days. Most women experience a menstrual cycle every 28 days.

In order to know your menstrual cycle, you must observe yourself for at least three consecutive months. Remember, the count begins on the first day of bleeding. For example, if you begin bleeding on December 10, you count that day as the first day of your menstrual cycle. You count each day of your menstrual flow and every day that follows until you begin bleeding again. If the next flow starts on January 7 (the 29th day), then you know that you have a 28-day menstrual cycle, which is the most common. Get a calendar and check it out!

Each month at the beginning of your cycle, an ovum, or egg, begins to ripen in the ovary. When the egg is ripe, it pushes its way through the walls of the ovary and enters the Fallopian tube. The process of the mature egg leaving the ovary is called "ovulation." Your fertile period is within 24–48 hours of this event. It is during these hours, if all is normal, that you can become pregnant. (See drawing.)

Ovulation normally occurs in midcycle, approximately 14 days *before* your next menstrual flow begins. An easy formula to remember in order to determine your time of ovulation is 14 days plus or minus two days before your bleeding begins.

For the woman whose menstrual cycle started December 10

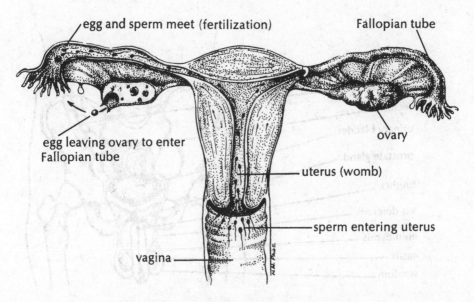

egg and sperm meet (fertilization)

Fallopian tube

egg leaving ovary to enter
Fallopian tube

ovary

uterus (womb)

sperm entering uterus

vagina

The Female Reproductive System—Conception

and ended January 6, ovulation was around December 23. If she had engaged in sexual intercourse within that period without using birth control, and if everything else was normal, she probably would have become pregnant.

Many women experience signs of ovulation. Some have slight spotting. Some experience discharge or a feeling that they are having a discharge. Some women's sexual desire appears to be higher. Many have no signs whatsoever.

You must observe your body carefully to know approximately when you ovulate. It is most important to know your fertility period if you wish to become or avoid getting pregnant.

An orgasm during the sex act is not related to your ability to become pregnant. This is probably what the "old folks" meant when they said, "Now that you have started menstruation you don't have to do anything. All a man has to do is lean on you, and you will get pregnant."

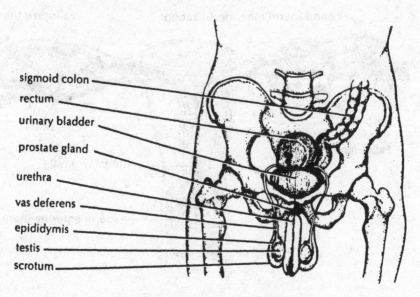

sigmoid colon
rectum
urinary bladder
prostate gland
urethra
vas deferens
epididymis
testis
scrotum

The Male Reproductive System

If conception does not take place, the egg dies, and the womb, which was preparing to receive and nourish the egg, sheds its lining as blood about 14 days later.

Events in the male are quite different.

The sperm, which under a microscope look like tadpoles, are produced in the testes of a healthy male at the rate of about one hundred million per day. From the testes, housed in the scrotum, the sperm begins a long journey. It is stored temporarily in a tube behind each testis called the epididymis. During ejaculation it travels through a continuation of these tubes, the vas deferens, which joins the seminal vesicles, two pockets located between the bladder and rectum. From here the sperm passes into the ejaculatory ducts, then into the urethra, and is expelled through the penis.

The outpouring of a fluid secreted by the seminal vesicle and the prostate gland during the sex act sweeps the stored sperm into the vagina.

The sperm of a healthy male may live 30–48 hours in the vagina, uterus, or Fallopian tubes of a healthy female. This may be the major reason for the high failure rate of the rhythm birth-control method, wherein sexual intercourse is recommended only during the "safe period." This period is calculated to extend from about seven days after menstrual bleeding ceases to about ten days before it resumes.

After the sperm are deposited in the vagina, they move in a swimming motion through the womb and into the Fallopian tubes. If ovulation has occurred in the female and the egg is waiting in the tube, one of the sperm will penetrate the egg, and it is in that moment of union that conception takes place. This is the beginning of the making of a baby.

2

The Black Father

Few people realize the anxieties newly expectant black fathers experience. Some suffer anxieties because of social and economic pressures; some because of concern for their wife and baby. Some feel that the pregnancy has proved their virility and suffer anxieties because of their eagerness to see what they have produced. A small number claim they suffer pregnancy-related symptoms such as morning sickness, unusual food cravings, and labor pains. While most are able to weather the storm, many experience extreme difficulties.

James had just finished college when his wife became pregnant with their first child. Shortly after the pregnancy began, his wife almost suffered a miscarriage and had to stop working for the duration of the pregnancy. But she was not eligible for unemployment compensation. James could not find a job in his field or any other field that paid an adequate salary and had to resort to unemployment benefits. Even though James was a brilliant student and a strong person, the pressures of unemployment and the concern for his wife caused him a great emotional strain. As a result, at the age of twenty-eight, James suffered severe simulated heart attacks.

Leonard and Betty were still in school and unmarried when Betty told him that she had missed her second period. Leonard began to look for a job. He was refused employment because he was either underqualified or overqualified. Or he was too great a risk because of the possibility of his leaving the job to return to college. After six months of a humiliating search Leonard dropped out of school and out of sight, even though he loved Betty and wanted the baby. His inability to be a "man" frustrated him, so that he felt the only way out was to run.

Most men are concerned about the health of their unborn children. To avoid letting this get you down, consider your own health and that of the expectant mother first. If both of you are healthy, if she is within the span of the recommended childbearing age and seeing a physician regularly, chances are the baby will be healthy. Should you have any lingering doubts, tests are now available that can detect many genetic disorders in an unborn child.

You should also be concerned about your health as an expectant father. Take care of your body by eating balanced meals, getting sufficient rest, and seeing your physician for your regular checkup. Tell your doctor if you are anxious about medical problems such as sickle cell anemia, hypertension (high blood pressure), and diabetes. It is important for you to tell the doctor and your wife if you have had a history of syphilis, gonorrhea, or drug usage.

If unemployment or low income is a cause for concern, don't allow it to interfere with your relationship with your wife. She, too, is undergoing a mental and physical strain. Whether this is her first or fifth pregnancy, she needs your help and understanding.

A pregnant woman tires easily and is sometimes nervous and irritable. She may also experience depression and may not desire you sexually. Some women are advised by their doctors to cease sexual intercourse after a certain stage in their pregnancy. If this is true in your wife's case, help her follow the instructions. This does not mean that you should not respond to her feminine appeal. On the contrary, she needs to know now, more than ever, that she is important to you.

Some hospitals allow the father to stay with the mother during labor. If this is a practice at the hospital where your baby will be born, it may be comforting to your wife to have you with her. If you wish to be present for the delivery, you should discuss this with your wife and her doctor beforehand, because some women are shy in certain situations.

You can further assist her by making sure the other children, if any, are in good hands while she is confined. If you are able to see that the hospital bill, baby's necessities, and living quarters are in satisfactory order, this will be an additional help in setting her mind at ease.

It would also be helpful if you as well as the new mother read materials on infant care before the baby arrives. You will then be able to aid her in taking care of the infant during those first hard months.

No matter what stigma the broader society has put on the black man as a father, we all know that every man is proud of his ability to procreate. Even though the black man has had many difficulties in shouldering the responsibility of fatherhood financially, he can provide the love and leadership needed in rearing a child. You can begin your role as a loving, guiding father now by being considerate of your wife before your child is born.

Some men feel their responsibility as father is satisfied as long as they provide economic security for their children. Some feel a father is only responsible for disciplining the children, and others that they are only responsible when a male child is involved, for whom a male image must be provided. What, then, is the role of the black father?

John returned home. He had been away for three days without contacting his wife and family. When he opened the door he found Sally, a known lesbian, talking with his wife. John told Sally that he did not allow half men in his house and asked her to leave. She replied, "What do you mean, your house? Your rent ain't paid and you haven't been around for days. Your baby is sick and you couldn't be found nowhere. You are the poorest excuse for a man I have ever seen. Why, I take good care of my woman and her children. They never have to look beyond me for love or money. I keep them well fed, well dressed, and give them plenty of spending money. You ain't no father to these children. When is the last time you gave them a dime? Why, if I was no more man than you, my woman would have left me a long time ago." John angrily responded, "If you think you are more man than me, zip down your pants and let's see who's got the most."

John and Sally were confusing John's virility and his ability to procreate with his role as a father. Men of all colors confuse these terms. Perhaps it would be worthwhile to give the definition of each.

VIRILITY: Manhood. Having the nature, properties, and qualities of an adult male; capable of functioning as a male in copulation.

PROCREATOR (often confused with father): A man who generates or produces an offspring. The person who begets.

FATHER: A male parent who acknowledges his responsibility for a child. One to whom family affection and respect are due.

If all men worked to be ideal fathers, would we eventually have a utopian society? That is a difficult question to answer. Yet many attribute the problems of the black community to the "absent" or "negligent" black male. Does the black man default by choice? Some men appear on statistics as absent because of institutional confinement or military service, others as negligent because of alcoholism, drug addiction, or inability to find suitable employment.

Studies indicate that the black man who has been classified as an "absent" or "negligent" father is not happy with his situation and would rather be with his wife and children. However, many such men have developed the ability to cover their true feelings by pretending that (1) they never really wanted children; (2) they dislike the mother of their children; or (3) to be a good father, one must be satisfied with one woman, which they find impossible.

Before considering your role as a father, you must understand your attitude toward yourself. If you are not satisfied with yourself as a person, you will not be able to share yourself with your off-spring, who is an extension of you. Economic deprivation and political subjugation have aided greatly in preventing the black man from feeling whole, but you must begin to recognize this. You must recognize this as a brainwashing method to frustrate the black man socially. Be aware. Don't frustrate yourself and your family. Set up your own realistic value system and take advantage of your special qualities. Don't worry about "keeping up with the Joneses," and you will succeed in feeling whole.

Your role as a father is based upon your ability to love and teach your children. It is your responsibility to learn and understand the system you live in so that you will be able to teach your children how to live better within that system and increase their self-esteem. Understanding the system is really not as difficult as it may seem. To understand the system one need not know all the answers, but one *must* know where to find the answers. That is, be able to tell your child *who* to see; *what* to do; *where* to go; *when* to do something; *why* it must be done that certain way; *how* to handle a problem. The core to understanding the system is who, what, where, when, why, and how.

Helping your child develop self-esteem begins at home. If you make negative statements to your child about him or black people in general, the child will associate blackness with inferiority. How often have you heard the statement "Act your age and not your

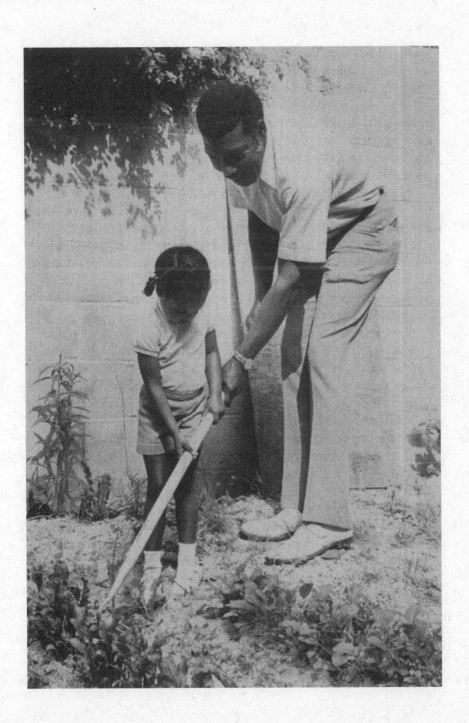

color"? What does this tell your child? It tells him that when he acts in any manner that is not Anglo-Saxon (white) and therefore right, he is acting unacceptably and only blacks act unacceptably.

It is your responsibility as a father to stress to the child his innate good qualities. Educate him on the contributions blacks have made to the world in music, science, mathematics, sports, and other fields. Motivate and encourage your child to learn the truth and achieve.

Always act in a manner that you would wish your child to imitate. If you use profanity, mistreat your black woman, have no respect for your property and that of others, spend money unwisely, your child will observe and pick up these undesirable traits. Never say to him, "Do as I say and not as I do." You are his example and a child's learning begins by imitating you. Until he understands or is introduced to religious teachings, *you* are his "supreme being."

A large number of black children seldom hear words of praise or love from their fathers. You must show your child that you love him and are proud of him. You must talk with him without always scolding or criticizing him. Many men withhold affection from their wives and children because they have been taught to believe that showing affection is not manly. Don't make that mistake. A child, male or female, needs affection. Children also need to know that you have love and respect for their mother.

Never tell a child that "things are rough" because of him. That burden is extremely difficult for the child to handle. A child must feel that his parents love, want, and enjoy him. Before he is born, he is secure within his mother's womb, and all his needs are satisfied. Perhaps this security before birth contributes to his ability to develop so rapidly during the first year of life.

If you, as a father, teach your child how to live, as well as how to make a living, he will love and respect you regardless of your financial status. This does not mean that you must not seek

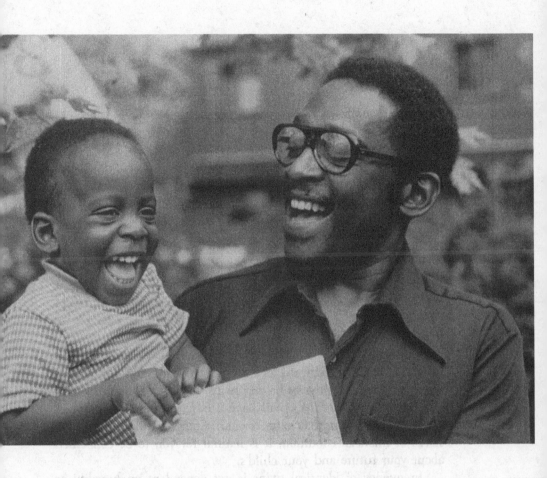

economic security for yourself and your family. However, it does mean that your economic level should not adversely influence your ability to be a father. Economic security is not the basis for love and respect. This has been proved by the many well-to-do families whose children receive many luxuries and too little love. Remember, the role of the father is not isolated from the role of the mother. These roles are complementary. The child needs both.

3

The Black Mother

Motherhood depends entirely on how you see life and yourself as a person. Many things may contribute to your ability to accept your pregnancy and motherhood, but nothing is as effective as self-respect and determination.

Pregnancy is not a difficult experience if you are a healthy woman, following your doctor's advice. It is natural for you to worry about such things as having twins, having a child born with birth defects, whether you will have a boy or a girl, the strain of delivery, and losing that extra weight. And, regardless of marital status or financial condition, it is natural for you to be concerned about your future and your child's.

Frequency of identical twins is not dependent on heredity or race. Frequency of nonidentical (fraternal) twins depends on: (a) heredity—history of twinning in maternal family; (b) race—(white: 1.05 per cent; black: 1.35 per cent of total births); (c) age—more frequently in older mothers; and (d) number of previous children—higher frequency in women with many children. Thirty percent of all twins born are identical twins.

If you are in good health and follow your doctor's advice, your baby will more than likely be born with no birth defects. Crossing your legs, folding your arms, laughing will not affect your delivery or your child's health, as some people believe.

Whether or not you suffer excessive pain in delivery depends upon many factors: size of the baby, position of the baby, size of your pelvis, length of labor, psychological preparation, and use of medication. The obstetrician normally measures your pelvic bone structure and, if he thinks it necessary for you to deliver by Caesarean section (see page 89), he will tell you long before you reach the delivery room.

Losing weight after delivery depends upon your prenatal habits. If you have eaten a balanced diet and exercised, you will probably have no problem losing extra weight.

Your body undergoes certain hormonal changes after conception. These changes may contribute to some differences in your personality. There are many moods of pregnancy. You may become more sensitive and irritable. You may become very quiet or very talkative. You may find yourself very tired one day and full of energy the next.

To become a mother does not excuse you from satisfying your husband's need for affection. You must be able to show him love and let him share in the care of the baby. It is a very demanding situation to be a wife and mother, but nature has given you the capacity to handle both roles.

The black infant usually receives a great deal of affection during his first year of life. The crisis begins when the mother loses trust and confidence in the child and in herself because she fails to recognize that there are certain behavior patterns common in black people. The average white infant has a slower pace of motor development and is less active than the average black infant. Society places greater value on the less active child, who supposedly sits quietly observing and learning his environment. The inference is that rapid motor development is unrelated to the infant's innate intelligence or intellectual potential. It is subtly suggested that the black child may possibly be hyperactive or

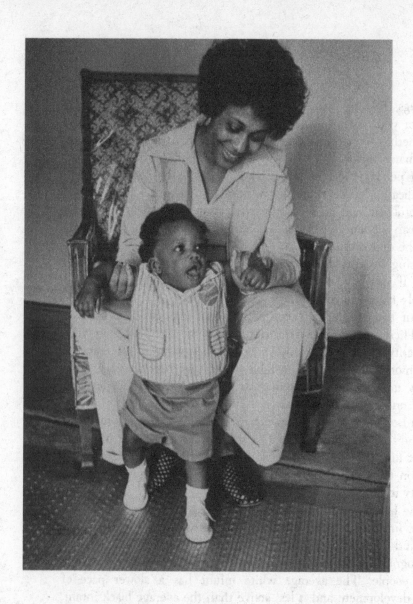

overly aggressive. Misguided by this suggestion, the black mother often holds back her affection and instead corrects, criticizes, and insults the child. She fears he may not meet the standard set up by the dominant society.

Because a child is very active and easily bored does not mean that he is hyperactive. Many of the things that are described as "hyperactive," such as walking early, getting into things, fidgeting, drumming with the fingers, shaking the legs while eating, chattering, are normal behavior in many black children.

If your child is a normal, active black child who is easily bored (not destructive or mentally retarded), you can channel his energy by providing him with learning activities, guidance, and love.

As a black mother, you must continue to give your child the love and attention you gave him during his first year of life. Do not smother him, but make him feel the security of love and family life.

When several black children were asked to describe an ideal mother, they all gave the same basic answers: an ideal mother shows love, communicates effectively, tries to understand, gives her children the chance to prove themselves before jumping to conclusions, scolds without violence, allows some privacy, shows and demands respect, is not overly protective yet shows authority and still remains a friend.

Are these children asking too much? A child who is comfortable and secure is willing to be obedient and cooperative. He is willing to learn and achieve. A child who knows that someone cares what happens to him also loves and cares.

The lessons of love and self-respect begin with you. It is your responsibility to teach your child where he came from, where he is, and where he must go. When you fail to face the problem of racism, you are not only crippling yourself, you are crippling your child and the black community. However, a child does not understand that "black is beautiful" simply because you tell him black is beautiful. Show him what you mean by pointing out the positive sides of blackness. The destruction of a people begins in the home.

It is your responsibility as a mother to point out your child's strengths and teach him the art of surviving. Encourage him. Help him plan his future. Guide him to useful and available jobs and careers. Help him to reach his own goal, not your unfulfilled goal.

Many black parents spend too much time telling their children what is "too hard" for them to do. Physics and chemistry are difficult if you say they are difficult. A child can learn chemistry just as easily as he can learn music. They both require discipline and concentration and they both require desire and effort. You direct your child's interest. You can give him a book to read just as easily as you can turn on the television for him to watch *Soul Train*.

As a parent, you are the manipulator of your child's environment. It does not matter that you are in a high- or low-income environment as much as it matters that you give your child the proper guidance to cope within his immediate environment and to expand into the dominant environment. Encourage him to learn the who, what, where, when, why, and how of the dominant environment so that he can function within it.

All children can learn, but each child has his own method of learning. Observe and understand your child's method and then help him reach his full potential.

Your activities, your mannerisms, your conversations, your attitudes have the greatest effect on your child's life. If you never read, your child will not read. If you criticize the black male, have no respect for yourself and other black people, your child will do likewise.

As a working black mother your problems will be compounded. You must make some additional efforts to direct the physical and mental growth of your child. You must strive to minimize any adverse effects the environment may have on the child because of your absence.

Your role as a mother extends beyond taking care of the child's physical needs. Almost anyone can feed, clothe, and clean a child. Most women can give birth to a child, but it takes much more to be a mother. As a black mother, you are the most precious gift to black progress.

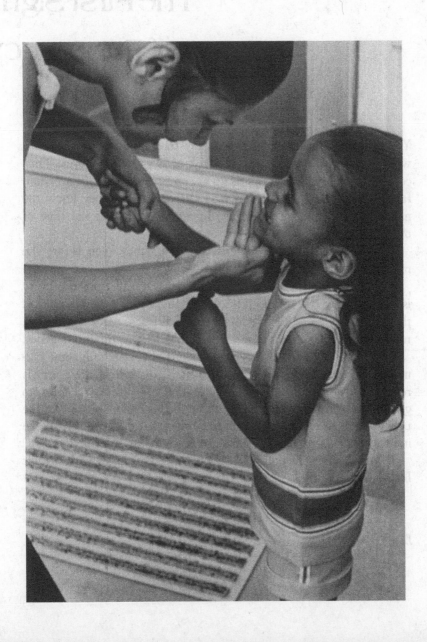

4

The First Signs of Pregnancy

You may have heard older people say that they can tell when a woman becomes pregnant by the look of her skin and eyes. They contend that pregnant women, upon conception, produce a certain facial glow. There are women who also claim that they knew the moment they conceived by the response they felt at the time of orgasm.

Can a woman make a diagnosis of pregnancy even before she misses her menstrual flow?

Conception takes place when the egg released from the ovary is fertilized by the sperm. The sex of the child is determined at that time, as well as all its genetic characteristics. After conception, nothing can change the sex of the child or the inherited genes.

Although millions of sperm bombard the egg, only one normally penetrates. The moment this occurs, the tail of the sperm is released. The fertilized egg divides and the embryo begins to grow. The embryo moves slowly through the Fallopian tube to the uterus. After a week of growth and travel, it attaches itself to the inner wall of the uterus, where a protective cover is formed.

Most women are not able to detect these changes within their bodies.

We say "most women" because some claim that they can. Some men also claim that they recognize the moment they procreate life. However, none of these claims has been scientifically substantiated.

As a rule breasts become enlarged and sometimes heavier immediately after ovulation or prior to the menstrual flow. When conception has taken place, the breasts become larger and heavier and the nipples grow and change to a darker shade. Blood vessels begin to enlarge, which causes a tingling sensation in the nipples. For some women this is the first sign of pregnancy.

Other signs are a suddenly increased desire to sleep, frequent urination, and increased amounts of saliva.

The most common sign is the absence of the menstrual flow or an irregular menstrual flow (pink or spotty bleeding). Some women also experience a thick, white, sticky discharge soon after their missed menstrual flow. Others experience nausea and vomiting as early as the second week of pregnancy.

All of the above are considered "presumptive symptoms" of pregnancy. Many women experience all or some of them when they fear pregnancy, desire pregnancy, or are suffering an undiagnosed illness. Although these signs are not reliable, they should not be ignored.

A doctor can give you a more accurate diagnosis through examination after you have missed your second period. You can also submit to a laboratory pregnancy test or check your basal body temperature. (See below.) Such tests are about 95 per cent accurate, but their results are still categorized as probable.

Pregnancy Tests

One of the most common tests used to determine pregnancy about two weeks after the missed menstrual flow is the immunological urine test.

This method tests for the presence of chorionic gonadotropin, a hormone produced by the placenta, which is formed only during pregnancy. The first morning urine is used for this test, which can be completed while the patient is still in the doctor's office.

The vaginal smear test may also detect pregnancy through hormonal changes. Here the doctor uses a cotton-tipped applicator to release the vaginal cells. This procedure tests the characteristics of progesterone, the female hormone, which is normally enhanced in pregnancy. This test, however, is very inaccurate and is rarely used.

The basal body temperature test, described below, is fairly reliable and may be done by you. The test is practiced by women who seek pregnancy or prefer the rhythm method of birth control. To verify pregnancy, use this procedure for at least four weeks following ovulation.

The test is based on the fact that a woman's basal body temperature is usually below 98° before ovulation. It rises between four-tenths and six-tenths of a degree after ovulation and remains at that level if pregnancy has occurred. If pregnancy has not occurred, the body temperature drops back to a temperature below 98°.

For this method to be effective, you must take your temperature every morning before rising, eating, drinking, talking, or smoking. Keep a thermometer by your bedside. You must keep the thermometer in your mouth for at least five minutes. If the temperature reading is consistently higher than 98° at least two weeks after your missed period, chances are that you are pregnant. Drugs, infections, alcohol, colds, or restless nights can, however, affect your body temperature and cause the reading to change. Take this into consideration when you use this method.

Your doctor can also prescribe a hormone to diagnose pregnancy. If menstruation does not occur within a certain period after the hormone has been taken, pregnancy is likely to exist.

Later Signs of Pregnancy

After the end of the third month, the lower portion of your abdomen begins to protrude and becomes very firm. Later, you can feel the fetus through the abdomen. A fluttering, known as "quickening," may be felt in the uterus. Quickening is the first perception of fetal movements, and is first noted from the eighteenth to the twentieth week of pregnancy.

Fetal movement, a definite sign of pregnancy, is felt between the fourth and fifth month, as is the fetal heartbeat upon examination by your doctor. The heartbeat can be heard by anyone about the seventh month, and is about twice as fast as your own. Do not be alarmed. This is normal.

Another way of detecting pregnancy is by X-ray examination, which, because of possible harm from radiation, is rarely used. It is highly recommended that you seek medical attention as soon as you suspect pregnancy. Many women put off prenatal care because of embarrassment, financial difficulties, or fear. Some believe that nature will provide proper prenatal care. The health of your baby means more than ten fingers and toes, all limbs, no outstanding abnormalities, and a pretty face. Lack of prenatal care and insufficient diet can prevent the brain from developing to its full potential, along with affecting a number of other important growth factors.

Prenatal care is a necessity. Your child's health is at stake. Your own health is at stake. Do not hesitate!

5

Selecting a Doctor

Who should guide you in your pregnancy? How should you select a doctor?

Whether you seek a family doctor or a specialist in obstetrics and gynecology depends largely on your family circumstances and where you live. In many countries, including the United States, midwives are trained to handle normal prenatal patients as well as uncomplicated deliveries. You may wish to use a midwife. If she is unable to handle your pregnancy, she will recommend a competent physician.

Today there are less than three maternal deaths to every ten thousand births, compared to sixty deaths to every ten thousand births before obstetrics and gynecology became a specialty.

While the competence of the doctor is a primary concern in making a selection, it is not the only one. You should also have respect for your doctor. Likewise, your doctor should respect you as an individual. Some women select and respect their doctor solely on the basis of race.

Mrs. Samson was examined by a young black doctor at the county hospital. The doctor told her that she had cancer, and removal of the uterus was recommended. Mrs. Samson replied, "I was born with my uterus and I shall die with my uterus." The doctor, recognizing the danger of such a decision, asked an older black doctor to check Mrs. Samson. The doctor examined her and made the same recommendation. Her reply again was, "I was born with my uterus, I shall die with my uterus." Finally, they called in the chairman of the department, who was also black. He made the same recommendation, but Mrs. Samson again refused. Hearing the doctors plead with the patient, a young white medical student walked over to her and said, "If you don't let them remove your uterus, you are going to die." Mrs. Samson replied, "Yes, sir, doctor. I'll let them do it." When the doctors asked her what made her change her mind, she replied, "Well, that white doctor said I must let you do it so I guess you were right."

Mrs. Samson is a victim of a widespread syndrome—if it's white it's right. Blacks caught up in this syndrome have been taught to associate blackness with incompetence and therefore feel themselves and other blacks inferior. In essence, they lack self-respect.

Is there an advantage to a black in having a black doctor?

Lillie Mae grew up in a basically middle-class environment. She attended predominantly white schools and churches and lived in a predominantly white neighborhood. When she became pregnant she felt that she could only get good medical care outside of her race. Lillie Mae had several scars on her body from childhood diseases. She did not drink, smoke, or take drugs. Nevertheless, when the doctor examined her, he asked her how long she had been on heroin, how often she had suffered infections such as syphilis or gonorrhea. She again felt stings of insult when he assumed that she was not married and would probably want an abortion. Finally, he asked her for her Medicaid number. No matter how she responded, the doctor remained oblivious to her answers. Lillie Mae might have saved herself from such insults

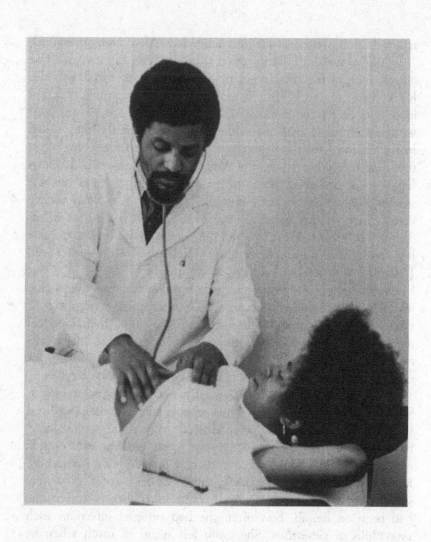

and humiliations had she sought medical care from a competent physician who did not stereotype his patients—one who could respect his patients as individuals regardless of their color or ethnic background.

When selecting your doctor, here are a few things you should consider:

A specialist in obstetrics and gynecology is trained in methods of prenatal care, labor and delivery, post-partum care, and diseases and problems of women. After completing a number of years in specialized training he is certified by the American College of Obstetricians and Gynecologists.

A specialist may cost a little more than a general or family practitioner.

A specialist will usually prove more skillful and experienced in obstetrical and gynecological care.

A general or family practitioner, if you and your family have been seeing him over a long period, knows you better.

Your family practitioner could recommend a competent obstetrician should a problem arise in your pregnancy.

A doctor of your own race will have a better understanding of your cultural background, of your fears and beliefs.

A doctor of your own race will more easily recognize and distinguish important environmental and genetic factors that relate to the individual patient.

A doctor of your own race has more experience with black patients and is therefore better able to recognize those problems that are peculiar to black women.

A doctor of your own race would be less likely to make assumptions about you based on color.

You must feel comfortable with your doctor. Whatever doctor you select, your first concern should be his competence as it relates to your present medical needs. Medical care goes far beyond checking your physical problems. You must strive to be healthy. A healthy pregnancy and a healthy baby begin with healthy parents, both physically and emotionally.

6

Visiting the Doctor

If this is your first visit to a doctor, he will ask a number of questions concerning your last menstrual flow, your past pregnancies, if any, and your family history.

A complete physical examination will follow. It should focus on the breast, abdominal, and pelvic structures. First, you are weighed, your blood pressure is measured, and a sample of your blood drawn. The blood test will enable the doctor to know your blood count, your blood type, and your Rh factor. It will also determine if syphilis is present. He will take a sample of your urine to check for an abnormally high blood-sugar level and the possibility of a urinary infection.

The doctor examines you vaginally (1) to determine the size of your uterus and your birth channel to ascertain if you are able to have a normal delivery; (2) to check for softening; and (3) to check for intermittent contractions. A Pap smear will be done to test for cancer and another smear to test for infections.

The doctor will then advise you of the procedure he will follow throughout your pregnancy. He will ask you to see him every three or four weeks during the first eight months and at least once a week during your last month of pregnancy.

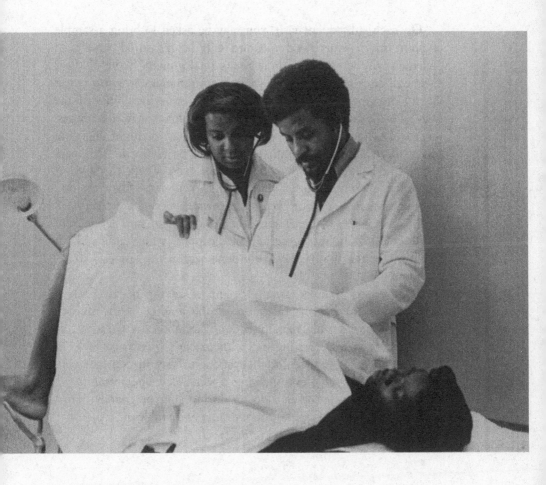

He will tell you when to expect your baby, based upon the information you have given him concerning your last normal menstrual flow. Delivery usually occurs about 280 days from the first day of your last period, the time needed for the baby to develop fully. He will discuss with you, among other things, the care of your body, activities permitted, diet, drugs, medicines, smoking, alcohol, travel, and sexual intercourse.

On each subsequent visit, you may be asked to bring a sample of your urine, your blood pressure will be measured, and your abdomen will be examined to evaluate fetal growth. Some of these visits will also include further vaginal examinations to get a better idea of the growth of the baby and to determine the ability of the baby's head to pass through the pelvis. Sometimes it may be necessary to ascertain how close you are to labor. If slight bleeding occurs after a vaginal examination, do not be alarmed. This happens. You should tell your doctor, however. Keep all of your scheduled appointments as faithfully as you can. They are important in managing your pregnancy toward an easier delivery.

In some cases, it is necessary for the doctor to start labor prior to the 280 days by giving certain medications, which also make it faster and easier. This is normally done within the last two weeks of the pregnancy.

Inducement of labor usually occurs when the doctor finds it necessary for the health and safety of the mother or the unborn child. In most cases of labor induction, the mother is either a diabetic (see page 61) or suffering with toxemia (see page 60). In these instances, it is wise for the patient to stay in constant contact with the doctor, never missing a scheduled appointment.

You will see a lot of your doctor during your pregnancy. Trust him! Don't hesitate to call him if you suspect a problem.

7

Taking Care of
Your Body

Many women are concerned about weight gain during pregnancy. They should be. Women who neglect their bodies during pregnancy will lose their physical attractiveness and may also experience other conditions such as varicose veins, stretch marks, increased waistline, sagging breasts, obesity, and heart disease. How can you overcome or avoid these problems? Take care of your body.

You will naturally gain weight during pregnancy, but this gain is manageable. The weight you gain because of overeating is not lost after delivery. You lose only the weight of the fetus, the amniotic fluid, and the placenta. Use the average weight gain of about twenty-five pounds as a guide. If you gain excessive weight over a very short period of time and your hands become puffy, your face rather full, and your feet swollen, you must see your doctor immediately, for you most likely have toxemia, a condition that can be harmful to you and your baby (see page 60).

STRETCH MARKS are lines that may occur on the abdominal skin as pregnancy advances. It is recommended that you avoid rapid weight gain as a measure against stretch marks. Many women wash their lower stomach area with cold water, dry it, and massage it gently with cocoa butter, olive oil, or cold cream. The effectiveness of this treatment has not been proved.

VARICOSE VEINS normally do not occur in the first pregnancy. Many believe this condition to be hereditary. Varicosity is the swelling of the veins in the legs and thighs. Pain in the varicose veins is a sign of phlebitis, an inflammation complicated by the varicose veins. If you have this tendency, keep your weight to a minimum. The condition can be aggravated by poor circulation, long periods of standing, and the weight of the baby. If you are concerned about varicose veins, you should wear elastic stockings. Discuss the best kind of support with your doctor.

Exercise your legs and elevate them for periods of time in the course of the day.

BREAST CARE is needed not only to avoid sagging and mastitis (breast infection) but also to condition your nipples for successful nursing. The first step toward breast care is a good maternity-nursing bra. If you have some old bras, cut a hole in the nipple area. Condition your nipples for nursing by washing them with a mild soap and water every morning after the sixth month. Rinse afterward with cold water and gently massage with a towel. If they become too hard, rub with petroleum jelly or cocoa butter. Around the fourth month the nipples may drain. If the drainage is excessive, cover the nipples. If the fluid remains on the nipples or if the nipples crack, wash them as often as necessary with clear boiled water cooled to lukewarm. Report this condition to your doctor.

TEETH. You should see your dentist as soon as your pregnancy is confirmed. Be sure to let him know that you are pregnant, since inflammation of the gums is common in pregnancy.

SKIN. Many women notice changes in their skin during pregnancy. Some experience darkened areas on their cheeks and forehead. All experience coloration around the nipples and a brown line which extends from the navel to the pelvis. This condition will disappear shortly after delivery. There is no need for extra care.

CLEANLINESS is of great importance. If you are accustomed to tub baths, you may continue to take them for the first few months as long as you are careful not to slip. It is advisable to sponge-bath or shower during the last few months.

DOUCHES. Many women douche after sexual intercourse. Douching should be avoided during pregnancy unless prescribed by your doctor.

BOWELS. If you eat a balanced diet and drink plenty of fluids, you should not have any problems with your bowels. Always remember to wipe away from the vagina after a bowel movement to avoid infections.

MEDICATION. During pregnancy do not use *any medication,* not even for a common cold or headache, without consulting your doctor. If you were on medication before becoming pregnant, let your doctor know. Some medications are harmful to your unborn child. For example, tetracycline taken during pregnancy is known to cause the child to have dark (gray) teeth.

SEXUAL INTERCOURSE during pregnancy may be permissible and safe until four weeks before the delivery date (not later, for fear of ruptured membranes) unless there is a history of miscarriages. In that case, intercourse must be stopped or restricted early in the pregnancy, based upon your doctor's recommendation.

In taking care of your body during pregnancy you should also rely on common sense. You need not stop living or become an invalid simply because you are pregnant. You should not overexert yourself either.

The ten commandments for a pregnant woman are:

1. See your doctor and dentist regularly and follow their advice.
2. Avoid contact with toxic chemicals or persons with infectious or contagious diseases.
3. Eat a balanced diet.

Taking Care of Your Body 35

4. Exercise daily but do not overexert yourself.

5. Get enough rest.

6. Avoid long periods of sitting or standing.

7. Get plenty of fresh air and sunshine. Don't become a hermit.

8. Dress comfortably and wear safe shoes.

9. Never take any medication before discussing it with your doctor.

10. Know the danger signs of pregnancy (see pages 64–66) and call your doctor.

Follow these rules to an easier delivery and a healthy baby.

8

That Important Diet

Christine was pregnant with her second child. She said that her first delivery was the worst experience in her life and she had no intention of suffering again. She therefore gathered "clean dirt" (dirt found at least one inch below the ground surface) to include in her daily diet. She had been told the "clean dirt" would make delivery almost painless because it would allow the baby to "slide out." Ellen ate a box of dry laundry starch every day for the same reason. She also wanted an easy delivery.

To include such items in your diet, whether you are pregnant or not, is very harmful. Both will cause chronic constipation, loss of appetite, and other complications, especially anemia or low blood count.

Many black women include excessive amounts of salt and pork in their diets. These may lead to toxemia and hypertension (see pages 60–61). If not treated promptly, toxemia can result in convulsions and even death, and hypertension or a stroke.

Another item often included in the diet of pregnant black women is ice—in the form of ice cubes or refrigerator frost. Many learn to like the taste and feel of ice. Others eat it because they have been erroneously told that it prevents heartburn. The expectant mother with a large ice diet can become anemic or suffer liver damage because this practice interferes with the consumption of nutritious, well-balanced meals.

An undernourished mother may give birth to a small, physically weak infant; her baby will probably suffer from anemia and most likely join the ranks of the slow learners at school age. The brain cells of a child before birth and during the first six years of life can be permanently damaged if the mother and child do not eat the proper foods. The health of your baby is largely determined by you, before and after conception.

If you are concerned about delivery, you might bear in mind that labor is easier for healthy persons, and you will most likely remain healthy if you follow an adequate prenatal diet. Your ability to breast-feed will also be far greater and your baby healthier if you follow a good diet during pregnancy.

Normally, the obstetrician will give you a supply of vitamins and minerals to use throughout your pregnancy as a supplement to your diet. You must take them as prescribed.

Most people eat according to their incomes. The higher the income the better their ability to eat well-balanced meals. Lower-income people usually include an excessive amount of carbohydrates. Such items as potatoes, sweets, and other fattening foods are cheaper. A high-carbohydrate diet may be filling and fattening but it does not provide the necessary amounts of proteins, iron, and vitamins. Drinking at least one quart (four 8-ounce glasses) of milk a day or eating cheese will help greatly to achieve a balanced diet. Milk is rich in nutrients; it contains proteins, minerals, vitamins, and calories.

Many black women find it difficult to drink four glasses of milk each day because if often causes gas and diarrhea. In fact, it has been discovered that the inability to drink large amounts of milk is fairly common in adults generally. Yet, many dieticians insist upon milk for children, senior citizens, and pregnant women.

Only the human animal feels that he should be contrary to nature and drink milk as an adult.

If milk is a problem for you, decrease its consumption or eliminate it from your diet. Eat more eggs, fish, and meats for your proteins instead. You can get calcium by eating green and leafy vegetables.

There are certain foods that should be re-evaluated in the black community. Two of these foods are sardines and collard greens.

Because these two items are looked upon as "poor man's food" or "soul food," their nutritional value is often lost to us.

Nutritionists normally recommend that a pregnant woman increase her intake of proteins, calcium, and carbohydrates, along with vitamins A and C. Lets compare whole cow's milk to sardines and collard greens to see how nutritious they are:

	Calories	Proteins	Carbohydrates	Calcium	Iron	Vitamins A	C
Milk							
(1 cup)	166	9	12	285	0.1	390	2
Sardines—							
(1 3-oz. can)	180	22	1	367	2.5	190	0
Collard greens							
(1 cup)	75	7	14	473	3.0	14,400	84

Sardines and collard greens also provide thiamine, riboflavin, and niacin. Although sardines may not provide much vitamin C, collard greens provide 84 mgs., whereas milk only provides 2 mgs. If you are on a low-sodium diet, however, sardines should be avoided.

The following is a list of nutrients found in foods that are common in the black community. Your doctor can give you a list of nutritional requirements for a pregnant woman. You can then figure out your own personal needs based on your weight and height.

	Calo-ries	Pro-teins	Carbo-hydrates	Cal-cium	Iron	Vitamins A	Vitamins C
Chicken, fried							
breast	215	24	0	10	1.1	60	0
leg	245	27	0	13	1.8	220	0
Pork chops (1)	260	16	0	8	2.2	0	0
Hamburger (1)	245	21	0	9	2.7	30	0
Grits (1 cup)	120	3	27	2	0.7	scant	0
Rice (1 cup)	200	4	44	13	0.5	0	0
Potatoes (1 cup) mashed with milk and butter	230	3	28	45	1.0	470	16
Sweet potato (1)							
boiled	200	2	36	44	1.0	8970	24
candied	295	2	60	65	1.6	11.030	17
Beans (1 cup)							
red	230	15	42	74	4.6	0	scant
lima	150	16	48	56	5.6	scant	scant
Blackeye peas (1 cup)	190	13	34	42	3.2	20	scant
Cabbage, cooked (1 cup)	30	2	9	78	0.8	150	53
Turnip greens (1 cup)	45	4	8	376	3.5	15,370	65
Peanut butter (1 T.)	90	4	3	12	0.4	0	0
Bread (1 slice) white	60	2	12	16	0.6	scant	scant
Eggs							
(1 boiled)	80	6.5	0.5	27	1.15	590	0
(1 scrambled)	110	7	1	51	1.1	690	0
Banana (1)	90	1	23	8	0.7	190	10
Orange (1)	70	1	18	63	0.3	290	66
Watermelon (1 slice)	60	2	12	16	0.6	scant	scant

You should not eat excessive amounts of foods rich in fats, sugars, and starches. These include bacon, fat meats, gravies, potatoes, mayonnaise, potato chips, spaghetti, rice, pies, cakes, candy, soft drinks, and popcorn. You should avoid highly seasoned and salted foods.

A simple guide to follow in meeting your daily dietary requirement is:

One quart of milk or milk substitutes
One cup of fruit or fruit juices
Two vegetables (one cup each)
One egg
One serving of cereal
Vitamins and minerals as prescribed by your doctor.

There has been much talk about the need for vitamin E. Of course it is needed, but not in overdoses. Few people suffer from vitamin E deficiency when their diets include green leafy vegetables, meats, eggs, nuts, vegetable oils, and other unsaturated fatty foods. The value of vitamin E in preventing varicose veins or mastitis (see page 34) or in ensuring an easier delivery, has not been proved.

If you already practice good dietary care, there is no need for you to make any special changes during pregnancy. Just remember, good eating habits mean a healthier and longer life for you and your child.

9

Black Folk Medicine, Superstitions, and Voodooism

There are many myths and superstitions about health, pregnancy, and child care in the black world. These attitudes have been categorized as "black folk medicine."

There are two forms of folk medicine: natural and magico-religious.

Natural folk medicine consists of the use of herbs, plants, minerals, and animal by-products in an attempt to cure illness. Some natural folk medicine practitioners use common sense and practical remedies; others may use very complicated and often harmful concoctions.

Magico-religious folk medicine includes occult practices such as voodoo and witchcraft, using charms, effigies, idols, holy words, and other mystic devices to cure medical problems. Diseases that are believed to be sent by evil powers are treated by spiritual intervention.

Many people believe that the practice of superstition and voodooism was the black man's first contribution to the medical world, but actually his first was a great physician, Imhotep, who lived in Egypt five thousand years ago. Some of his remedies are still used today. A group of European medical doctors recently made a study of the African witch doctor's inventory of natural remedies and concluded that a number of them have been incorporated into modern medicine.

Even when licensed doctors are available, people still use black folk remedies and charms to cure illnesses and ward off evil spirits. Though such beliefs are unfounded, occasional success, through coincidence, results in their continued acceptance.

Pregnancy

Here are several examples of folk beliefs.

Essie watched her son as he awkwardly played in the center of the room. She sadly explained that she had not seen a physician about his club foot because his condition was a result of her actions while she was carrying him. She and her sister were grocery shopping one day when they saw a stock clerk dragging around the store on his club foot. This struck her as the funniest sight she had ever seen. She held her stomach and laughed until she cried. She couldn't help herself. When her child was born a few months later, he, too, had a club foot. "I marked my son," she said, with tears in her eyes.

Louise ate strawberries almost every day of her pregnancy. Her daughter was born with a strawberry mark on her stomach. Juanita's baby was born with a scar resembling a dog on his neck because she had put her hand on her neck when told that her dog had bitten the newspaper carrier.

Many believe that if a pregnant woman is frightened and touches her stomach at the time of her fright, her child will be born with a birthmark that resembles the object of her fright. Other beliefs are that a woman should never fold her arms around her stomach or cross her legs while carrying a baby because these movements may cause the umbilical cord to wrap around the baby's neck and choke him. Some say that one can always tell the sex of a baby before it is born: if the baby is a girl, boys will give the pregnant woman much attention while girls will practically ignore her. The reverse is true if the child is a boy. Some also believe that a pregnant woman should rub her stomach daily with her dirty dishwashing water to insure an easy delivery.

Although none of these folk beliefs have been proven harmful, parents need not resort to them. If they are both healthy and the mother sees a doctor regularly and follows orders, their baby is more than likely to be born healthy.

Delivery

Many practitioners of black folk medicine believe that the mother's health is protected if no one sweeps under the bed where the birth takes place. Some insert cobwebs and soot mixed with sugar in the vaginal track to prevent hemorrhage after delivery. Others believe that if the afterbirth is late, the mother should stand over a pail of hot coals until she is completely smoked. Once the afterbirth has been released, they feel it should be either burned or buried to keep the mother from hemorrhaging or having other complications.

Breast milk can be dried by putting a needle in a broom straw and tying it around the mother's neck, according to some believers of folk medicine.

Much harm can result from some of these remedies. A new mother should be kept in a dust-free area, especially if she suffers from any respiratory problems. The cobweb, soot, and sugar remedy in the vagina could cause an infection. How many women are strong enough immediately after delivery to stand over a pail of hot coals?

The New Baby

In some cases, a child is not named until after the ninth day because of the belief that it may die if named before. In naming a child, it is thought that if the initials spell a word, the child will grow up to be wealthy. Other beliefs are: a smart or good child will die young; you will cause the death of an infant if you rock his cradle while empty; a pretty baby will grow to be an ugly adult and an ugly baby will become pretty; never allow an infant to look behind him, his eyes will cross; if you cut an infant's fingernails with scissors before he is a year old, he will grow up to be a thief; never carry a baby in a funeral procession before his first birthday if you wish him to live through his youth; a baby's hair should not be cut before his first birthday because it will make him weak; you should not measure a baby during the first year—to measure a baby is to measure his grave.

To protect a child fully from illness and evil spirits, the voodoo remedy is horehound, ash leaves, basil, and holy herbs mixed together in water and applied to the child's forehead in the form of a cross.

None of the above practices could really harm the child but are mentioned as examples of surviving superstitions.

There are countermeasures and medicines prescribed by folk practitioners for children to correct physical traits or cure illnesses. Some believe worms can be extracted from a child by rubbing his stomach with turpentine; or that a baby should always wear a band around his waist to make his back strong and allow him to sit up earlier; or that a navel hernia can be corrected by putting lard and powder on a piece of scorched cloth and tying it against the hernia with a band around the stomach to hold the burned cloth. The band is to be changed every other day, but the scorched cloth should not be tampered with. For some, a silver dollar placed over the hernia is equally effective. Many believers feel that hiccups can be cured by putting a straw on the baby's fontanelle (soft, pulsing area in the skull); chicken pox can be cured by taking the child to a henhouse and allowing the chickens to fly at him; mumps can be cured by rubbing the swollen areas with sardines; and measles can be cured by massaging the body with corn meal. A large number of practitioners believe that a dog's lick will cure a sore; fatback and a penny will extract glass from the foot; a boil can be dissolved by rubbing a dead person's hand over it three times; a common cold can be cured by placing an asafetida bag around the neck; a splinter in the hand should be removed and the splinter placed in one's hair to avoid ever getting another. Other believers say sweet oil dropped in the ear will cure an earache; kissing a dog's head will cure a cold sore; never pierce your ears or consent to surgery during dog days (forty days during late spring or early summer). For teething, some practitioners recommend that you cut off an unskinned rabbit's head, remove the brains, and rub the child's gum with the brains.

Obviously, the above list does not nearly exhaust the many folk cures and superstitions found in the black community.

These beliefs are not just shared by the poor or uneducated. They are quite often practiced among people of middle- and high-income levels. Although higher education seems to make one more skeptical, many college students and other people of learning have begun to seek the advice of palmists, spiritualists, root workers, and astrologists.

While most of these cures and beliefs are harmless, some are extremely dangerous and could cause permanent damage such as mental retardation and physical deformities. To be safe, consult your doctor, nurse, or pharmacist before using home cures.

10

Your New Appearance

Pregnant women have mixed emotions about their appearance during the long waiting period. Some feel fat and ugly, some feel more feminine, many tire of having to wear maternity clothes.

Most pregnant women normally buy a couple of nice maternity dresses and try to use as many of their regular clothes as possible. The working woman may buy four or five outfits to last through the working weeks.

While you are waiting, it is important for you to look well groomed. Many men think a woman is much more attractive when she is pregnant. Mr. Smith, who was seventy-two, would take his daily walk near a home for unwed mothers. His philosophy: "There is nothing lovelier than a pregnant woman."

The first rule in buying maternity wear is: buy styles that will suit you, and be sure they are well made and expandable enough to last you through your pregnancy. You don't have to spend a lot of money to look attractive. One simple method to enlarge your wardrobe is to purchase two or three maternity skirts or pairs of slacks and match them with a number of pretty shirts.

Genevieve and Carolyn were known as the best-dressed teach-

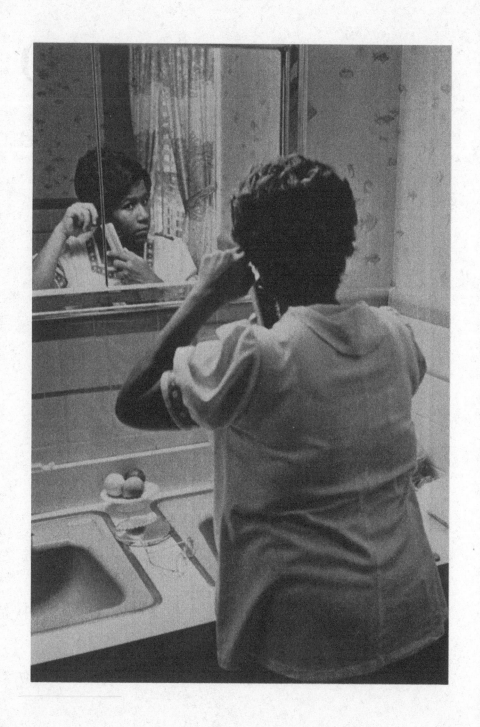

ers in their city's school system. Luckily they were never pregnant at the same time so they lent each other maternity clothes. It saved them money and they were still the "best dressed." Exchanging maternity wear with friends is a good money-saving practice.

Sewing maternity clothes is very easy. Even a beginner can handle it. There are many "quick to make" patterns on the market that offer a variety of fashionable outfits. Buy inexpensive materials that are easy to handle. Compare prices and buy discount or sales items.

You will need larger bras. Maternity bras are available and can be used after the baby is born and during the breast-feeding period as well. Two should be adequate.

A maternity girdle is only necessary if your doctor advises it, but you will need larger underpants and underslips.

You must wear shoes that can adequately support you and your extra weight. Narrow high heels, three-inch platforms, heels with bare backs or narrow straps are out. You cannot take the chance of slipping or falling, so confine yourself to low (not necessarily flat), closed-in shoes. Shoes with straps are sufficient as long as they fit closely and confine the heel.

Clothes are not the only thing that keep you attractive while you are waiting. If you are accustomed to applying make-up, continue to do so. Keep your hair and nails attractive.

Personal hygiene is a must while you are pregnant. In essence, keep on looking good while you are waiting. You don't have to exhaust your funds to do so.

11

The Mother's Activities

Many women believe that pregnancy naturally restricts their normal activities. This is far from the truth.

Most pregnant women continue to work unless their work involves an unfavorable environment. Discuss your job with your physician. Let him help you make the decision since it may involve your health and the health of your child. You should also discuss with your doctor your ability to continue your sexual activity.

You can travel while you are pregnant, by car, bus, train, airplane, or boat. Your travel should be based upon your physical strength and the availability of a licensed medical practitioner. Always consult your doctor when you plan long trips.

You can also continue most sports activities and other forms of exercise. Walking is one of the best exercises a pregnant woman can take. So why not take a walk every day?

Take only those exercises or participate in those activities that will not present the hazard of slipping or falling. How much you exercise depends largely upon how much you can handle. You must never exhaust yourself, and you must rest afterward. Never push, carry, or lift heavy or large objects.

The importance of posture cannot be overemphasized, since many women tend to let out their abdomen and curve their backs as the baby gets heavier. This habit is one of the main causes of lower back pain. You should avoid the swayback position by "thinking tall." Walk, sit, or stand with your shoulders up, and your chest and buttocks out. Don't curve your back.

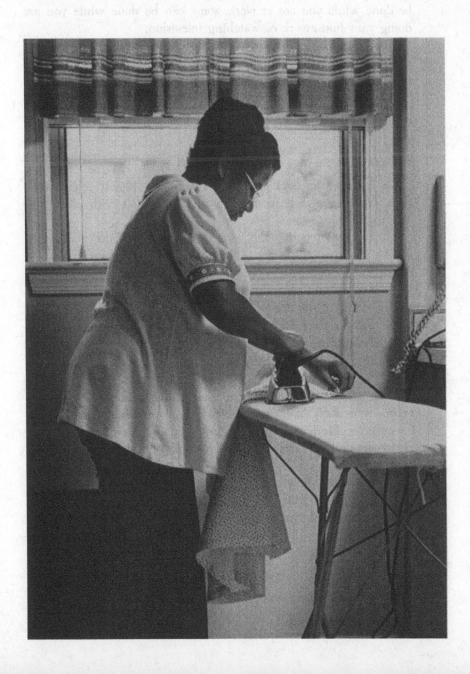

There are some special exercises that can be taken during pregnancy to help you have an easier delivery. They can also help you avoid backaches, pain in the legs, and poor circulation, and they can help later to restore your figure. Some of these exercises can be done while you are at work, some can be done while you are doing your housework or watching television.

To begin with, dress as comfortably as possible in a pair of shorts and loose top. You will need a pillow only when you do those exercises in which your head rests on the floor. The number of times you perform an exercise depends on your ability to handle it. But do not overexert yourself.

Exercises

1. Lie on your back and clench your fists. Slowly release your grip. This can also be done in a sitting position with your arms hanging by your sides.

2. Lie down with your arms to your sides. Raise your arms. Keep them up to the count of five. Now let them down slowly and relax.

3. Tighten up your shoulders and count to five. Release them slowly. This can be done while lying or sitting.

4. Lie on your back and tighten up your leg muscles. Raise your left leg slightly above the floor. Hold it up for a count of five. Now bring the leg down very slowly (count to ten). Relax. Do the same with the right leg.

The area of your body between the thighs is called the perineum. We don't have to emphasize how important that area is for delivery. Here are some exercises that will strengthen the perineum for delivery and help you regain your figure shortly after delivery.

1. Sit on the floor with the soles of your feet together. If you are unable to get your feet together, cross them at the ankles. In this position, push your right knee down to the floor with your

right hand. Hold the knee down to the count of five and release it. Do the same for the left knee, using the left hand. You can read, sew, or watch television while in this sitting position.

2. Lie on your back with your hands at your sides and your knees slightly elevated. Slowly raise your back and buttocks. Hold this position to the count of five. Relax.

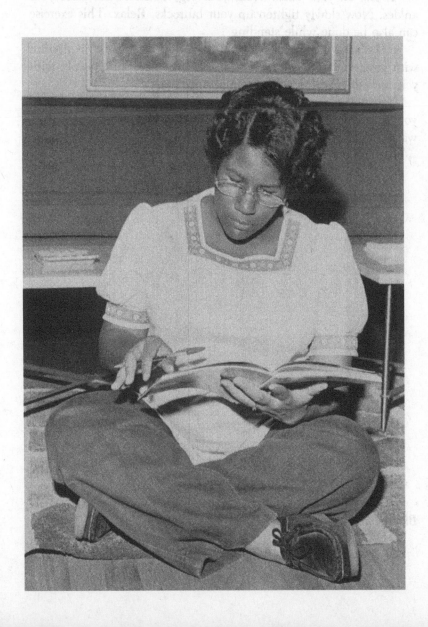

3. Lie on your back with your hands at your sides. Point your toes. Raise your right leg, without bending it, as high as possible. Count to five and take a deep breath. Now bring the leg down again. Do the same with the left leg.

4. Lie flat on your back. Arch your back as much as you can, and count to five. Now return to the flat position. Relax.

5. Lie on your back. With your legs outstretched, cross your ankles. Now slowly tighten up your buttocks. Relax. This exercise can also be done while standing.

6. Labor will be easier if you learn how to breathe in rhythm with your contractions. You can practice by breathing deeply with your mouth closed. Count to ten and exhale.

You will discover that these exercises are easy and will not tire you. Exercise daily for an easier delivery and a good figure afterward.

12

Minor Problems in Pregnancy

There are certain discomforts in every pregnancy. If this is your first pregnancy, you will probably worry about things you have heard. If your anxieties are based upon fear of pain or death, please be assured that the pain will be tolerable and the risk of death almost nonexistent if you have received proper medical attention.

If you are concerned about added weight, remember that if you eat and exercise as directed, the weight you gain will only be temporary. If you fear the role of motherhood, dismiss that concern. This anxiety ordinarily disappears as your natural motherly instinct develops. In most cases anticipated difficulties never materialize. Should minor problems arise they are generally overcome with patience and determination.

If you are excessively anxious, ask your doctor to help you analyze your fears. Friends who have experienced pregnancy and motherhood may also be helpful.

NAUSEA AND VOMITING. Many women complain of nausea and vomiting (morning sickness) during the first couple of months of their pregnancy. This condition is usually felt in the morning, but is sometimes experienced throughout the day. Quite often it is emotional in origin. Unless this condition is severe, you shouldn't let it disturb you. It usually disappears before or by the end of the fourth month. You should eat smaller amounts of food more frequently to help lessen the discomfort. If you find that certain foods bring about nausea and vomiting, avoid them. Rest also provides relief.

CONSTIPATION. Constipation is the inability to relieve your bowels after more than two days, or the passage of a very hard stool. You need not have a bowel movement every day. This complaint is more common among those women who have inadequate diets or who eat "clean dirt," clay, and dry laundry starch. The problem can be controlled by adjusting your daily diet to include plenty of green leafy vegetables, salads, fruits, cereals, and about eight full glasses of water. One of the most common problems among black women is that they don't drink enough water. Many say they don't like the taste and too often they take laxatives on their own. Do *not* use a laxative without consulting your doctor. Walking is a good exercise to help lessen constipation.

HEMORRHOIDS. Hemorrhoids, or "piles," may appear or increase during pregnancy. They are caused by the increased pressure of the uterus on the veins in the lower rectum and, of course, they are worsened by constipation. Pain and swelling of the hemorrhoids can be relieved by medication prescribed by your doctor.

BLADDER PROBLEMS. Urinary frequency, the urge to urinate, and occasional "accidents" are common complaints of the pregnant woman. The problem is usually caused by the pressure of the uterus against the bladder as well as increased blood flow to the kidneys. Cutting back on coffee and tea and not drinking alcohol can sometimes relieve this problem. Normally you will return to your usual urinary habits after delivery. Always tell your doctor if you are experiencing severe discomfort or pain when you urinate.

BACKACHE. Most women suffer a small degree of pain in the lower back during pregnancy, especially if they have strained themselves by lifting heavy objects, bending too often, or walking too much. Pain in the back may also be a result of unsuitable shoes, poor posture, or fatigue. If your backache is persistent or extremely painful while sitting, lying, or standing, tell your doctor.

HEARTBURN. This is a burning sensation in the chest with an acidlike taste in the mouth. Heartburn is a common complaint in pregnancy and can generally be relieved by drinking milk. If you are unable to drink an eight-ounce glass of milk, check with your doctor for suitable medication. Eating crushed ice cubes will not remedy the condition. Do not use baking soda or any other formula before talking with your doctor.

FAINTING. Fainting is not uncommon at the beginning of pregnancy. Some women consider it a first sign of pregnancy, although there is no scientific validity to this claim. Fainting or dizziness should be reported to the doctor at once.

CRAVINGS (PICA). Many people consider cravings for certain foods, cornstarch, or dirt a common symptom of pregnancy. To date, no one has been able to relate the two scientifically. It is believed that most cravings are promoted by old wives tales, and are actually emotional desires.

VARICOSE VEINS. See page 34.

INCREASED SALIVATION. An uncomfortable increase of saliva is sometimes noted during pregnancy. If this is true in your case, let your doctor know and he will try to correct the condition.

TIREDNESS AND SLEEPINESS. It is not uncommon for a woman to complain of her inability to stay awake or of constant fatigue during the first four months of pregnancy. If you feel tired and sleepy, go ahead and sleep if circumstances permit. This condition usually subsides after the fourth month.

VAGINAL DISCHARGE. This is not unusual during the last few months of pregnancy. If there is an excessive amount of thick secretion accompanied by itching, report it to your doctor. If the discharge is thin and pale yellow, don't worry unless it is excessive. Do not douche unless advised to do so by your doctor.

HEADACHE. This is a common complaint early in pregnancy. Do not take medication before consulting your doctor. Normally, the headaches stop by the end of the fourth month.

SKIN AND HAIR PROBLEMS. Some women experience skin discoloration, which is sometimes very prominent about the face. It is frequently referred to as the "mark of pregnancy." The breast, nipples, and midline may also become darker. Stretch lines on the abdomen sometimes appear and the hands become red. A number of tiny pimples may appear on the face. Some women claim their skin is smoother and healthier looking during pregnancy. Some complain that their hair becomes dry, more coarse, breaks off or falls out, whereas others say that their hair grows faster. Give your hair and skin the same treatment during pregnancy that you do ordinarily. If you should have problems, rest assured that your hair and skin will return to normal after delivery.

BREATHING PROBLEMS. Shortness of breath is not uncommon as the pregnancy advances. Rest more often during this period. If you have difficulty sleeping, lie on your side with your head and shoulders resting on one or two pillows. As the infant moves into the pelvis for delivery, the condition subsides. If you experience great difficulty breathing, you should, of course, tell your doctor.

MUSCLE CRAMPS. As your body gets heavier, you may experience cramps in your thighs and lower leg muscles. The weight of the baby sometimes contributes to poor circulation in these areas. Some muscle cramps can result from calcium deficiency, but most often they are attributed to lack of exercise and sleeping on the back. Tell your doctor if you are having muscle cramps.

NASAL STUFFINESS. Postnasal drip or a feeling of stuffiness in the nose is common. In pregnancy this condition may be relieved by using a vaporizer. If the condition persists, seek the help of your doctor. Do not take any medication.

TEETH PROBLEMS. In some women gums become inflamed and bleed at the slightest touch. Small round, purplish-red spots may also appear on gums. This condition may worsen as the pregnancy matures. Use a mouthwash. If the condition continues, see your dentist. If you did not see a dentist early in your pregnancy, be sure to see one at this time. The changes in your mouth are due to hormonal changes in your body. One common condition is called a "pregnancy tumor," which is a small bump in the mouth. Of course, there are old wives' tales regarding teeth and pregnancy. Some women complain that they lost their teeth after having children. Your teeth will suffer only if you neglect them.

Most of the discomforts of pregnancy can be handled or relieved. Many will disappear after the first few months. Some women experience most of the difficulties mentioned while others experience very few or none at all.

13

Medical Problems Common to the Black Pregnant Woman

Certain serious illnesses are especially associated with the black community, and pregnant women should be on the alert for them.

TOXEMIA. This disease is commonly found in the young black female during her first pregnancy. It generally occurs in the last few months and begins with a rapid weight gain and swelling of the face, hands, and feet. Blood pressure steadily goes up, and severe headaches and chest pains are experienced. If these symptoms are ignored, convulsions, coma, or even death may result.

The cause of toxemia is unknown, but present studies point to diet as an important factor. If your doctor gives you a specific diet during your pregnancy, you should follow it. Undoubtedly, you have heard people say: "The doctor gave me a list of foods to eat, but there is nothing on it that I like and I can't starve to death," or "The doctor told me not to eat salt, but this little bit won't hurt," or "I've got to have just one of these pig's feet. I've been eating them all of my life and they haven't killed me yet."

HYPERTENSION. Commonly known as "high blood pressure," hypertension is among the leading causes of death in the black community. It is not yet clear what part diet plays in this disease, but most authorities believe that salt, fatty foods, and early obesity (overweight) are important factors, along with kidney diseases.

Hypertension often begins in the very young and may progress rapidly. In a pregnant woman, hypertension is frequently mistaken for toxemia, because the symptoms are similar: swollen feet, face, and hands and very high blood pressure. Such cases require emergency care. The baby's and mother's lives can be in jeopardy.

ANEMIA is a deficiency in the oxygen-carrying capacity of the blood. The condition has various causes, including poor diet.

The concentration of blood hemoglobin and red blood cells is often lower during pregnancy. This is an important reason for adding supplementary vitamins and iron to your diet.

Common symptoms of anemia are paleness in the palms of the hands and the conjunctiva (pink part of the eyelid), lack of energy, excessive need for sleep, and shortness of breath.

It is important that you watch for the signs of anemia while you are pregnant because this condition interferes with the oxygen supply to the fetus. As a result, the child may be born smaller than average, his brain may not mature, or he may develop heart problems.

DIABETES. Diabetes is hereditary. The trait may be latent and not appear until influenced by conditions such as pregnancy or excessive weight gain. A very large baby at birth is an indication of a diabetic trait in the mother, requiring careful evaluation for possible onset of overt diabetes. An adult is more likely to get the disease than a child; a woman is more likely to get it than a man.

Some of the symptoms for this disease are: frequent urination in large amounts; constant thirst; weight loss with an increased intake of food; drowsiness and fatigue; chronic infections; inability to have sexual intercourse (male impotence); itching of the genitals and skin; blurred vision and other eye problems.

If any of these symptoms should become apparent, tell your doctor. Some women develop the disease during pregnancy and more often than not return to normal after the delivery. Doctors refer to them as "gestational diabetics"; but they are treated as full diabetics because the effects are equally devastating in both. Generally, on this level the disease can be controlled by diet alone, but in some cases insulin is required.

Diabetic women who do not follow their doctor's orders usually miscarry, deliver dead babies (stillbirth), or give birth to large infants with many difficulties.

Diabetes cannot be cured but it can be controlled.

A diabetic woman is always delivered before term to prevent stillbirth, frequently by Caesarean section (see page 89) if induction of labor fails. The baby is normally treated in the same manner as a premature infant, even though it is very large. The controlled diabetic has fewer complications at delivery and the infant is healthier. An uncontrolled diabetic mother usually gives birth to a very large infant who may have hyaline membrane disease (a covering on the lungs that causes suffocation); or an extremely large infant with a round reddish face and swollen cheeks, low blood sugar, and problems of the central nervous system.

The problems of pregnancy as they may affect a diabetic are not necessarily complex, but they do demand careful attention. You must stay on an adequate but low-salt diet and take your insulin.

SICKLE CELL ANEMIA. Sickle cell anemia is a disease of the blood caused by an abnormal hemoglobin—the oxygen-carrying part of the blood—which bends, or "sickles," the red blood cell when the oxygen concentration in the blood is lowered. A person who has the sickle cell *trait* is normal but has the capacity to pass sickle cell anemia to his children if he mates with a person who has the trait or the disease. You should have your blood tested for sickle cell before marriage if you plan to have children.

A woman with the sickle cell anemia *trait* usually has a normal pregnancy and delivery. However, during the last few weeks of her pregnancy she may develop urinary-tract infections.

If a woman with the sickle cell anemia *disease* becomes pregnant, the disease usually becomes more intense. Pain is frequent and lung diseases are common, as are toxemia, infections in the womb, and swelling of the veins. At least half of the sickle cell disease patients miscarry or deliver stillborn babies or babies who die some time during the first few weeks of life.

A person with this disease requires close medical observation and careful treatment at the time of delivery.

14

Pregnancy Danger Signs

There are several danger signs of pregnancy that should be *reported immediately to your doctor,* should you experience any of them. They might indicate serious problems that could endanger your life or the life of your unborn infant.

VAGINAL BLEEDING. Some women spot during the first few months of pregnancy. This should be reported. If you experience bleeding or pains in the lower abdomen area that resemble menstrual cramps around the time you normally have your periods, or at any other time, go to bed, abstain from sexual intercourse, and call your doctor.

SWELLING. Swelling of the face, feet, ankles, or fingers, especially after a night's rest, is an indication that abnormal fluid is accumulating. Call your doctor.

EXTREME REDUCTION OF URINE. This could be serious if you suddenly have difficulty discharging your urine even though you have been drinking your usual amounts of liquid. Call your doctor.

FLUID LEAKAGE FROM VAGINA. A sudden uncontrollable leakage of clear fluid from the vaginal area could be a sign of early or term labor. Call your doctor.

HEADACHES. Frequent or persistent headaches should be reported to your doctor.

VOMITING. Persistent vomiting (*unlike* morning sickness) must be reported to your doctor.

CONVULSIONS (FITS). This is similar to an attack of epilepsy. Its symptoms are violent contractions of the neck muscles, usually jerking the head back, rolling of the eyes, and hands extended or held in a tight fist. If you respond to the danger signs of pregnancy by reporting them to your doctor, you are not likely to experience convulsions. However, should you suffer convulsions, you should be taken to your nearest emergency treatment center immediately.

DIZZINESS OR BLURRING OF VISION. This condition may be a result of fluid retention. In addition, some women also experience mental confusion and see spots before their eyes. These signs take some time to develop and will not be experienced if you have been seeing your doctor regularly and reporting all unusual conditions.

PAIN IN THE ABDOMEN. Soreness in the abdomen and alternating contractions may be normal. Constant severe pain or repeated pelvic or abdominal cramps must be reported to your doctor.

CHILLS AND FEVER. A viral or a bacterial infection of the reproductive or urinary tract usually causes chills and fever and requires medical attention without delay.

WEAKNESS AND INCREASE IN HEARTBEAT. Frequent heartbeats (palpitations) and fainting are not uncommon in pregnancy. This condition, however, should not be combined with an occurrence of violent pain in the lower abdomen accompanied by fainting— probably an ectopic pregnancy (pregnancy in the Fallopian tube). Ectopic pregnancy is extremely dangerous and, therefore, these symptoms require prompt action. See your doctor immediately.

RAPID WEIGHT GAIN. If you have gained more than ten pounds without increasing your food intake within two to four weeks, let your doctor know. Don't think that the weight gain is unimportant or fear the doctor may reprimand you.

SEVERE CONSTIPATION. If you have been eating a balanced diet and drinking an adequate amount of fluids, but have not had a normal bowel movement for five or more days, call your doctor.

The importance of consulting your doctor promptly on any of the above conditions cannot be overemphasized. If your doctor is not available for any reason, go to your nearest medical emergency center.

15

Pregnancy and Drug Abuse

Flossie felt happy. She had just delivered a three-pound-nine-ounce boy in the eighth month of her pregnancy. In the past, Flossie had experienced three miscarriages. Her doctor said that she smoked too heavily, but Flossie could not break the habit. During this pregnancy she had cut down to half a pack a day. Was this "small," early delivery the most Flossie could hope for? Would the child grow to be a healthy and strong adult?

Tina smoked reefers (marijuana) during the first two months of pregnancy, eventually moved on to sniffing "coke" (cocaine) and then to shooting up heroin. She became addicted and needed drugs daily. With the aid of friends she continued her habit even while she was in the hospital for delivery. Her daughter was born an addict. Within a few hours the baby was crying excessively. By the end of her first day of life, she began trembling and scratching herself. On the second day she started vomiting and could not be fed. Finally she suffered convulsions.

The two-day-old infant was experiencing heroin-withdrawal symptoms. Tina was able to get friends to supply her habit, but her daughter had no friends. Did she deserve this agony as her start in life?

Every human being has the right to be born of healthy parents; to be born to parents who want him or her; to be properly delivered, fed, and immunized as an infant; to be reared in a stable home (not merely a house) where love and tender care abound; to grow up in a home and neighborhood as free as possible from high concentrations of toxic chemicals and physical and environmental hazards; to grow up in an atmosphere of recognized spiritual values and practices. This is particularly true now that birth-control methods and abortions are freely available.

Is a child born to a mother who is a heavy smoker, dope addict, or alcoholic given these basic rights?

Even those parents who give their children up after birth want to see them healthy and productive. As a parent, you may best foster that desire by keeping your body healthy and free of preventable diseases.

The pregnant woman should avoid use of *all* drugs, especially those harmful to the central nervous system of the fetus. Drug addiction in pregnancy causes withdrawal symptoms in the newborn along with development of other serious abnormalities which have not yet been fully evaluated. Alcohol is believed to be harmful to the fetus, although there are no specific data to support this belief. Cigarette smoking is associated with a smaller baby at birth. It is also believed to cause serious lung disorders such as bronchitis and pneumonia if one or both parents smoke around the infant during the first year of life. Infants with these symptoms are more susceptible to SIDS (Sudden Infant Death Syndrome). Danger from narcotics is much greater than from cigarettes or alcohol.

No matter how superhuman you may feel, the use of narcotics leads to an intense emotional and physical dependence. No unsupervised drug user can avoid this risk. Once a person becomes addicted, changes occur in his behavior, work, love life, and ability to reason. Improper drug use can also lead to undernourishment, lower disease resistance, and inadequate functioning of vital organs. Misuse of depressant drugs blunts the senses of the mother and prevents the full development of the brains of the infant within the mother's womb, causing mental deficiency and, in some cases, physical handicaps.

Few things are as tragic as an addicted infant. Even though most are able to survive the crises of birth because of improved medical care, many are so heavily addicted that they convulse within a few hours after birth and die. Death sometimes occurs because the mother denies recent use of drugs, preventing proper medical attention for the newborn. You *must* tell the hospital if you have used drugs. You should do whatever is necessary to give your child a normal, healthy start in life.

The best advice to a potential mother regarding the use of addictive drugs, alcohol, or cigarettes is: *don't*. If you are already "hooked," tell your doctor immediately. He will help you to withdraw as quickly and safely as possible.

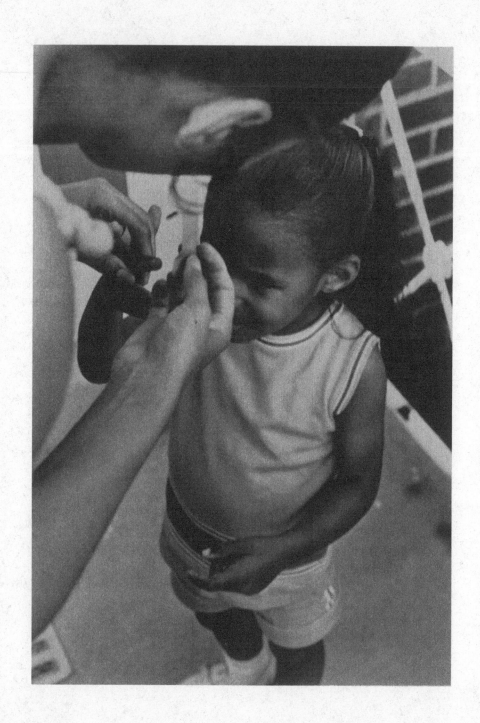

Part Two

Infant and Child Care

16

Selecting Your Child's Doctor

Before you deliver, you should select a pediatrician for your baby. A pediatrician is a doctor specializing in the care of children from birth to twelve or so.

Most hospitals include a pediatrician on the delivery team to check your baby at birth, but you may have one of your own choice. Whatever the case, your child should be thoroughly examined.

Select your child's doctor carefully. Your child will be reared in a competitive world. He will be exposed to a number of complex social and economic situations. You need a doctor who will treat your child's physical illnesses and will also have an interest in him as an individual; a doctor your child will be able to relate to and have confidence in. He must also be able to deal with the child's emotional problems. It is important to find such a doctor at birth because he is likely to play an important role in your child's life for many years.

At birth, the doctor weighs, measures, and examines your infant, and checks for birthmarks, birth defects, and rashes. He visits you in the hospital and gives you a summary of his findings as well

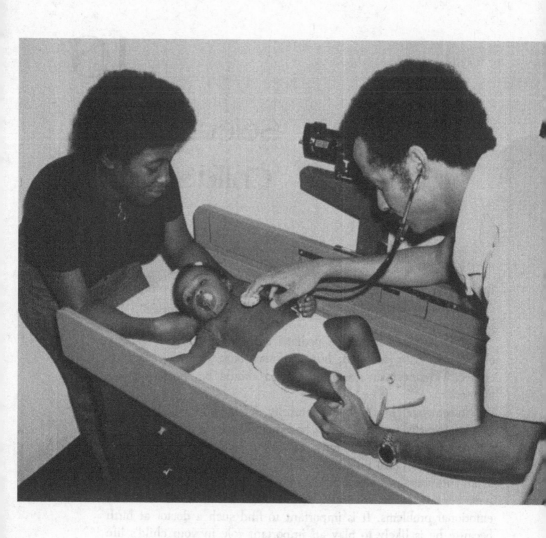

as advice on feeding methods. He may also give you a "guide for new mothers" that includes common problems of the newborn.

Your child should have regular visits to the doctor, especially during his first year. There are many things on which the doctor must advise you, including the baby's diet changes, weight gain, eyes, hearing, feet, and his motor development.

Call your doctor whenever you have reason to be concerned. It is strongly recommended that you find a competent physician who will not only manage your child's health care but who is also aware of and can relate to his cultural needs. This is important because many blacks grow to adulthood before ever seeing a black doctor.

Tony was eight when he became seriously ill. He had had some common childhood diseases and had been immunized at the clinic, but he had never been taken to a doctor. One of his mother's co-workers recommended an extremely competent and well-recognized pediatrician. Everything ran smoothly for Tony's first visit to a doctor's office until the doctor walked in and said, "Hello, Tony, I'm Doctor Jones." Tony began to scream and fight to get out. "You are not a doctor," he said, "you are a black man and there are no black doctors. A nigger can't do nothing right so you know he can't be a doctor."

At eight, Tony had already learned self-hate. Did this black child learn that black is inferior from his parents, his friends, the mass media, or relatives?

To help you and your child accept the competence of black physicians, consider that in 1893 Dr. Daniel Hale Williams performed one of the first open-heart operations; in 1940 Dr. Charles R. Drew developed a practical method of preserving human blood (the blood bank) that has permitted doctors all over the world to save countless lives; Dr. Hildrus Poindexter and Dr. W. Montague Cobb, both consultants for this book, are world-renowned physicians—Dr. Poindexter for his ingenious method of stamping out malaria and other tropical diseases in Africa and the Philippines during World War II, and Dr. Cobb for his achievements in the fields of anatomy and anthropology. These are just a few of the many contributions blacks have made in medicine.

17

Labor and Delivery

Getting Ready

You should spend your last few weeks preparing for the delivery. Many hospitals require that you preregister at least six weeks before your infant is due (preferably much earlier) to allow them time to have your bed reserved, your records organized, identification tags made, and a number of other things done to insure good patient care.

Think about naming your infant before you reach the hospital. Consider both male and female names. Select carefully, as his name will stay with him for the rest of his life. Avoid giving your son a female name and your daughter a male name. It is equally important to know the meanings of the names you select, and watch out for initials that spell words. There are a number of books available that include lists of American names or names from Africa. Two recommended books are *The Book of African Names*, as told by Chief Osuntoki, by the *Drum and Spear* staff, and *The New Age Baby Name Book* by Sue Browder.

Check to see that all the items your baby needs are in order. If you plan to use a formula, have on hand at least six eight-ounce bottles with nipples and two four-ounce bottles with nipples, a bottle brush, and a large pot for sterilizing the bottles and nipples.

The baby's clothing should include at least three dozen washable diapers or six dozen disposable diapers, three pairs of rubber pants, three nightgowns, four undershirts, a sweater, two blankets, three receiving blankets, two water-resistant mattress pads, and two crib sheets. If you plan to use a bassinet, a pillowcase can be used as a sheet.

Some cotton, baby oil or petroleum jelly, cotton tips, baby pins, baby lotion, two bath towels, and a basin or baby tub should also be included in your layette.

If you are unable to provide a bedroom for your new baby, a specific area of your house should be set aside for the infant's care and rest. The area should be large enough for a portable crib because the average black baby is unable to stay in a bassinet longer than two months.

Your baggage should be packed about two weeks before the expected delivery date. It should include:

Mother
    Clothes to wear home
    Two nightgowns
    One bathrobe
    One pair of slippers
    Two nursing bras
    One sanitary belt
    Cosmetics and toilet articles
    Personal telephone directory
    Pen and pad

Infant
    One nightgown
    One undershirt
    One receiving blanket and/or heavy blanket
    One pair of rubber pants
    Two diapers

Labor

Sometime during your last month of pregnancy, you may notice that your baby has dropped lower in the abdomen, which is known as "lightening." Once lightening has occurred, you may be able to breathe easier. If this is your first baby, you will probably deliver within three weeks. If you have had other children, lightening may not be observed before labor begins.

The hours you spend in labor depend mainly upon your age and the number of children you already have. If you are having your first child, you may labor for as much as fifteen hours. If you have had children before, you may labor for only six hours or less.

The signs of labor are:

1. Mild pains (contractions) in the lower abdomen and back. These pains will increase in force at a regular rate and can be timed by a clock. For example, you may note that at first the pain lasts for ten seconds and recurs every thirty to thirty-five minutes. If this is your first baby, you should call your doctor when these contractions come every five minutes. If you have had one or more children, call your doctor when the contractions are ten minutes apart.

2. A small amount of red or pink discharge may be seen. You may also have a bit of blood. If there is actual bleeding, you should go to the hospital immediately.

3. You may experience a sudden uncontrolled loss of water from the vagina that is clear and odorless. If the "water breakage" occurs, immediate hospitalization is recommended, regardless of presence or absence of contractions.

Do not eat solid foods once you recognize the signs of labor and are able to time your contractions. This is important, especially if you wish to receive anesthesia.

When you arrive at the hospital, tell the admissions office that you are in labor and give the name of your doctor. You will be given a general physical examination and taken to the labor suite until you are ready to deliver. During the time you are in the labor suite, your baby's heartbeat will be checked regularly, you may be given an enema, and the hair may be shaved from your pubic area. Your cervix will be checked periodically to ascertain the progress of labor. If necessary the doctor will give you a painkiller to help make labor easier. Once your baby is ready for delivery, you will be taken to the delivery room.

Delivery

You will normally wait no more than thirty minutes for your baby to arrive after you've reached the delivery room. You can help relieve the pains of labor by breathing with your contractions. Active bearing down with contractions will also assist the descent of the baby's head—after full dilation of the cervix is achieved. Ordinarily, anesthesia is not given until the infant's head has pushed through the dilated (opened) mouth of the uterus.

The doctor will use one of several safe methods to reduce your pain at the time of delivery. A common method is to give general anesthesia, which puts you to sleep for a short time. During this time the baby is delivered and the afterbirth (placenta and membranes) removed. This method of relief may pass a significant amount of the drug on to the infant, causing him to be less alert at birth.

Another common method is the use of regional anesthesia. The spinal block, which consists of injecting drugs in the spinal column, prevents pain below the waist. It allows you to remain conscious during the delivery. Post-delivery headaches are a side effect, however a similar method is the use of injections in the area around the spinal cord. These two methods have very little influence on the infant. However, they do require close observation of the mother after delivery as some women have toxic reactions from their use.

The paracervical block is another pain-relief method used at delivery: the mouth of the womb and the nerves that supply that area are anesthetized. Novocaine, injected in the vaginal area, is one of several drugs used to relieve the terminal pains of delivery. This method also allows you to stay awake during delivery with very little pain.

These are only a few of the anesthesias used during a normal delivery. Many women, however, elect to deliver without using any anesthesia. This is considered natural childbirth. The most common method used today is the Lamaze, which is based on various breathing exercises to relax the mother during labor. Both parents participate in a course of instruction consisting of both the breathing exercises and physical conditioning. If you are interested in natural childbirth, consult your doctor. He will tell you whether or not you are able to handle labor without anesthesia and where you can receive instruction.

If there is a need to perform an episiotomy for an easier delivery, you will be given a local anesthetic or any of those discussed above. An episiotomy is a small split made at the external opening of the vagina, when the vagina is unable to expand enough to allow the infant's head to pass without tearing the area. The cut is easily repaired by stitches that will melt away within a few days.

Your next move is to the recovery room. Your abdomen is massaged and examined to insure that all is well. After about one to two hours, you are taken to your room.

Your stay in the hospital varies according to you or your doctor. However long it is, be thankful, for you have just participated in one of life's greatest wonders.

Post Labor

Before you leave the hospital, your doctor and your baby's doctor will give you some specific instructions. Take notes.

Most doctors advise that you refrain from sexual intercourse for at least six weeks after delivery. Follow these instructions.

Your first few weeks at home may be tiring. Get as much rest as possible. If you want to exercise, talk it over with your doctor.

After the delivery, you will have a bloody and eventually a white creamy discharge. This should cease by the end of the six-week period.

For most women who don't breast-feed, menstruation returns within the first three months after delivery. A nursing mother, however, may not menstruate until after the infant has ceased nursing.

Bear in mind that menstruation may not be regular for many months after delivery. Do not assume that you won't become pregnant simply because you are nursing or not having regular menstrual periods. If you wish to avoid becoming pregnant again so soon, talk it over with your doctor.

A number of women complain of depression and anxiety shortly after delivery. "Baby blues" may be a result of hormonal changes—a return to normal. Whatever the cause, do not allow the blues to get you down. Your doctor, relatives, or friends may be able to help you. Talk with them.

Most obstetricians see their patients six weeks after the delivery to check if the body has returned to normal. They will also discuss family planning, and will advise you to see a physician at least twice a year for a general examination.

18

Characteristics of the Newborn

Janice had just delivered her first baby. She was overjoyed that she had delivered a healthy son, but she was concerned because the baby was covered with a thin white substance, his legs were drawn and wrinkled, and his puffy eyelids glued together by a heavy white substance.

Many women are disappointed when they see their newborn because they expect him to look like the month-old baby next door. Here is a brief description of a newborn baby:

Weight: The normal full-term male black infant weighs about seven pounds at birth. Females are somewhat lighter.

Length: The average length is 19–20 inches.

Head: The normal head circumference measures 13–14 inches, and usually seems large for the body. It may be round, lopsided, or elongated. There are two soft spots (fontanels) on the head. One is at the top center of the head and the other, at the back, is very small. You may notice the pulse-like movement of the fontanels, especially the one at the top of the head. The scalp may be loose.

Hair: The hair may be thick, thin, curly, or straight; or the newborn may appear bald, but in reality has thin lanugo, "baby hair."

Eyes: The eyelids may look puffy or the eyes slightly crossed. These conditions usually correct themselves. If the eyes are unusually crossed and remain so for more than six weeks, ask your pediatrician's advice, or take your infant to an ophthalmologist for possible corrective measures.

Skin: Most of the color will be on the ears. Some infants are hairy on the face and ears. Many black infants are born with dark or bluish spots (liver spots, medically referred to as Mongolian spots) that normally appear on the upper or lower back. These spots are caused by pigment in the

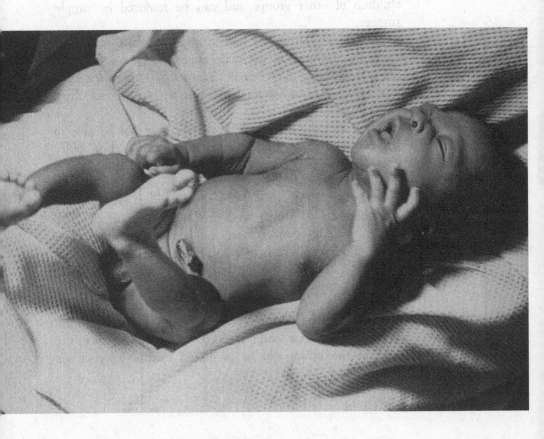

deeper layers of the skin. They are completely harmless and normally disappear by the time the child is five years old.

Hands: Some infants hold their fists tight, while others keep their palms open. The palms have very fine lines and the fingernails are thin. The skin on the hands is loose and the wrists are heavily creased. Extra fingers are more common in black infants than in white and can be removed by simple surgery.

Legs: The legs remain drawn and are somewhat short compared to the arms.

Feet: The skin is very loose and the feet appear to be flat. Extra toes are more common in black children than in children of other groups and can be removed by simple surgery.

Genitals: The vagina in the female and the penis, and especially the scrotum, in the male appear to be too large for the infant's body. The female infant may experience some white discharge and vaginal bleeding within the first three days.

Face: Who does the baby look like? You may not be able to tell because of the broad flat nose, receding chin, puffy eyes, and pudgy cheeks. The infant's personal features will be defined later.

Body: The neck is normally short, the shoulders are rounded, the abdomen is round, and the hips are narrow. The breasts may be swollen and the navel string tied. Evidence of an umbilical hernia (bulging) may not be present until after the navel string has dropped. If an umbilical hernia is present, it will usually close by the fourth or fifth year.

"What color will he eventually be?" is one of the first questions asked when a black child is born. Some believe that the "true" color of the infant can be predicted by the color of his ears. Others suggest it is the flesh around the fingernails and toenails.

Color should be of the least concern for new black parents. Genetic factors and black history make the range of color tone wide, regardless of the parents. We say "black is beautiful," but do we honestly believe this slogan if we continue to be concerned about the shades?

Hair is another major concern of black parents. It is said that straight hair in an infant means soft and fine hair later, and that curly hair will become extremely hard to manage, or "nappy."

Even though many attitudes have changed and we are not as brutal toward each other regarding the texture and length of hair since the natural hair styles, comments on "good" or "bad" hair are still present and need to be eliminated.

These are some of the erroneous beliefs passed along from one black generation to the next. Hair does not aid our ability to think or function. Its only function is to cover our head. So, whether hair is short, long, curly, hard to manage, or straight should be of little importance. Enjoy your child during the first year of his life. Don't worry about the texture of his hair and the color of his skin.

Too many of our present difficulties stem from the weight we put on matters over which we have no control. Skin color and hair texture fall into this category. They don't aid in the mental growth of the child. They don't help him to reach his potential. The standards we use to judge what is best are based upon the standards set by the ruling society. Although these standards have no basis in reality, they have done much to give black people a sense of inferiority. The media are the greatest promoters of this inferiority, through fashion magazines, movies, television, and beauty contests.

Your child is an extension of you. If you like the way you look, you will like the way your child looks. If you are unhappy with yourself, you will be unhappy with whatever physical traits the child inherits from you. If you are unhappy with yourself, don't take it out on your child. Don't teach him self-hate. Teach him self-love. Don't allow your neighbors, relatives, or friends to burden your child's life with a negative attitude. Stop them when they say, "Lord, his hair sure is gonna be nappy. Look how curly it is now."

Help your children to be proud of their inherited physical characteristics from the very beginning.

19

The First Days

The first few days of your baby's life will be difficult for both you and your baby. If you deliver at a hospital, you will be required to stay there from three to five days, depending on your health, your wishes, and your doctor's policy.

Immediately after delivery, the baby's skin is cleaned of its white covering, and his navel string (umbilical cord) is shortened. Some hospitals give vitamin K as an insurance against bleeding. Many check blood and urine for abnormalities and put a solution in the eyes to prevent eye infections. The baby is also weighed and measured.

Your baby's footprint and your fingerprints may be taken as a part of his birth registration and an identification bracelet will be placed on his arm.

Some hospitals provide facilities for the newborn to stay in the room with the mother, especially if the mother decides to breast-feed. Check with your doctor to see if this arrangement is possible at the hospital you will be using.

The average hospital places newborn infants in a nursery where they are cared for by nurses. They will bathe and change your infant and observe his bowel movements for regularity and color. The color of his skin will also be checked for any irregularities. As mentioned earlier, a pediatrician or a general practitioner will examine him on the first day.

Your infant will be brought to you for his daytime feedings. If you have chosen to breast-feed, you will find that you will not have milk immediately after delivery, but rather a yellowish liquid (colostrum), which will nourish him until the milk comes. Breast-feeding may be painful in the beginning, but you should persist because it has many advantages.

If you have chosen to bottle-feed your baby, his formula will be brought to you at the time of his feeding.

For the trip home, naturally you should dress him according to the weather—in warm clothing and wrapped in a heavy blanket if it is cold; otherwise, in lighter clothing and wrapped in a lightweight blanket.

You will probably be driven home from the hospital. Place your infant in a baby carrier for his protection.

Be sure that you get a birth certificate for your infant as soon as possible. He will need it when he begins school, or when he applies for a job or a driver's license.

You may wish to have someone at home with you for the first few days. Perhaps a relative or friend can help you get organized. Your baby's father can also be very helpful. Allow him to share completely in caring for the infant. He is capable of preparing bottles, feeding, and changing diapers, among other chores. Don't leave him out.

An infant cries when he is hungry, cold, hot, thirsty, tired, wet, uncomfortable, sick, or lonely. If you have taken care of all these needs and he continues to cry, check with your pediatrician.

You cannot spoil a newborn infant by treating him tenderly. Give him love and care from the very beginning, and he will give you love and respect in return.

20

The First Six Weeks – General Care of the Infant

The most critical time of life occurs at the beginning. A young plant is most vulnerable when its head just peeks out of the soil. Even the biggest and strongest animals are helpless when they are only a few weeks old. So it is with a child. During the first four weeks the infant makes his greatest adjustment from the protected warmth of his mother's body to the outside world.

The first day is, by far, the most critical of all. In medically unsupervised situations more deaths occur during the first twenty-four hours than during the next twenty years. For this reason, a pediatrician should be present shortly after delivery.

An infant's weight falls during the first week of life, but is regained around the tenth day. The length of time he spends in the nursery varies. Most normal full-term babies are discharged after three days unless a complication or an infection arises. Babies born by Caesarean section—that is, removed surgically from the mother's abdomen—are released after five days.

Prematurity

A premature infant is one who has had a gestational period of less than thirty-seven weeks. Prematurity and low birth weight usually occur together. In the United States, a low-birth-weight baby is one who weighs less than 5½ pounds. The average birth weight varies in different parts of the world.

Studies* show that 7 per cent of white live-born infants and

* Waldo E. Nelson, Victor C. Vaughan III, and R. James McKay, *Textbook of Pediatrics*, 10th ed. (Philadelphia: W. B. Saunders Co., 1975), p. 341.

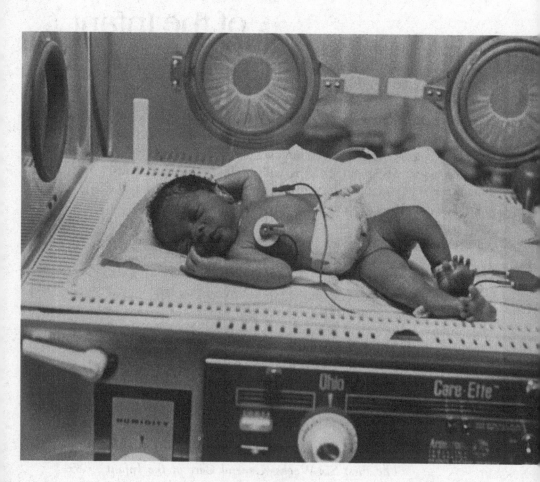

14 per cent of black infants weigh 5½ pounds or less. However, it is interesting to note that the death rate in the first four weeks of life is lower among black infants.

Prematurity and low birth weight are usually tied in with social conditions—lack of prenatal care, insufficient food intake by the mother, and overwork. Some common medical causes are: anemia, premature rupture of the membranes, toxemia, and multiple pregnancy (twins, triplets, etc.). Infants who are premature have an increased chance of developing diseases of the lung, eyes, and other organs. For example, jaundice and low blood sugar are seen more frequently in the premature infant, along with an increased incidence of congenital malformations.

The premature and low-birth-weight baby is carefully watched in the hospital nursery for complications and signs of disease and is not sent home until he reaches the weight of 5½ pounds. Prematurely born children usually catch up to other children in development by the time they are two or three years old.

Emotional Growth

It is easy for you to handle your child's physical growth. You feed him, you bathe him, you weigh him, you watch his limbs fill out. But his emotional growth is a little bit harder to handle and observe, but is equally important to his total development.

You must begin now by providing him with the best possible environment. This doesn't mean putting him in a large, expensive home with beautiful furnishings. It means clean and comfortable surroundings. It means protecting him against outside influences that may adversely affect his mental growth.

Your child's protection begins with you. The infant easily detects your anxieties and often responds by refusing to eat, by overeating, or with just plain fretfulness. You must handle your infant with sensitivity because your acceptance of him is essential.

Marian married a handsome, light-complexioned man. Her

sister married her husband's twin brother. When her sister's son was born, Marian commented that he was the "prettiest" baby she had ever seen. He had straight hair, light-colored skin, and big gray eyes. She was very excited about her own pregnancy one year later and anticipated a baby just like her sister's.

When Marian's baby son was shown to her, she asked the nurse to take him away because she was tired. She complained later to her husband about how ugly her son was. "He is not only black," she said, "his hair is going to be nappy. How could I have had such an ugly baby? Neither you nor I are black like that." Marian's husband was surprised at her reaction. "I think he is very handsome," he said. "In fact, he looks just like my mother."

Marian was never able to accept her son, and her son was aware of her displeasure and hurt by it.

If you allow your child's life to begin in an environment of rejection, he will behave negatively for the rest of his life.

The inherited traits of your child cannot be changed. The stress of birth is shared by you and your infant. His acceptance of being born is largely dependent upon the degree of satisfaction expressed by his parents and family from his earliest days.

Physical Care

SCHEDULING. If this is your first child, you may wish him to set his own schedule. Take note of the times he sleeps, eats, or lies awake, and help him keep this schedule. Be ready to feed him when he is ready to eat, bathe him when he first awakens in the morning, and enjoy him while he is awake.

If there are other children and you need to put your newborn on a schedule, you may have to wake him to feed him, allowing flexibility for the infant who may wish to eat more or less food, or sleep more or less hours.

Always remember to bathe your infant before you feed him since he will normally be sleepy after his meal.

HICCUPS. It is normal for young infants to hiccup. Usually the hiccups disappear within a few minutes.

VITAMINS. Your full-term infant will need supplemental vitamins. Some prepared formulas already contain the necessary vitamins. If the one you are using does not, ask your pediatrician to prescribe them separately. These vitamins are prepared commercially in syrup form, and can be placed in the formula or directly into the baby's mouth. If you use a dropper, place it in the cheek of the mouth or on the tongue, *never* in the back of the baby's mouth.

BOWEL MOVEMENT. Some of the questions pediatricians are asked most frequently concern the stool of a baby, which is different in appearance and consistency from that of an older child or adult. At first it is a sticky substance, dark green or black in color. After four days the "transitional" or "changing" stool appears, which is curdy and greenish or yellowish brown.

CONSTIPATION. Bear in mind that the consistency of the stool rather than its frequency is the criterion for assessing constipation. A constipated stool is firm and dry. So a child may have a bowel movement at regular intervals, but if the stool is firm and dry he is still considered constipated. Most infants have at least one stool daily, but some perfectly normal babies have a stool only every three to four days. In most babies constipation is due to dietary imbalances, which can be readily corrected. Do not use laxatives, enemas, or suppositories.

DIARRHEA. Here again the character of the stool rather than its frequency is the determining factor. The diarrheal stool is loose and very watery. Diarrhea in the infant can be caused by infectious bacterial organisms and can result in a high mortality rate. However, this type is rarely seen today because of improved medical care. Diarrhea can also be caused by viral infections.

In the first three weeks of life, overfeeding is the most likely cause of diarrheal stools. This type of diarrhea is relatively common, thanks to the anxiety of well-meaning parents. Formulas that are too condensed or have too high a concentration of sugar can also cause diarrhea. Most mild cases respond well to simple procedures such as decreasing or diluting the feedings. However, if there is no improvement, or if there is blood in the stool, get medical help.

COMFORT MAKERS. There are a number of ways in which babies may comfort themselves. These include thumb sucking or sucking a pacifier, hair twisting, or holding the end of the blanket. Some believe these habits satisfy the infant emotionally. Others view them as the infant's method of communicating certain needs or desires. For example, he may suck his thumb or do any of the above if he is hungry, tired, or sleepy. Hair twisting and blanket holding help some infants fall asleep.

It is believed by some researchers and mothers that infants who are breast-fed or fed with moderate-size holes in their bottles do not thumb suck.

Most people now believe that comfort devices used by infants and young children are normal. However, a physician or counselor should be consulted if a child uses them beyond six years of age.

CRYING. All babies cry. This is one of the earliest means of communicating.

You should form the habit of responding to your baby's needs promptly. This does not mean, however, that you must rush to his side as soon as he whimpers.

When your baby does cry, check to see if he is hungry, wet, cold or hot, or simply wanting attention before you assume that he is ill. Remember, some infants cry violently because they want to go to sleep. The important thing is to stay calm and not let your child sense anxiety on your part.

If a child is crying excessively, you should check his comfort. Are you overfeeding or underfeeding him? Is he being burped properly? Is there tension or noise in his environment?

If you are unable to determine specifically why he is crying, your infant is probably suffering from colic. If this is so, he will double up his arms and legs, his face will redden and his stomach will feel very hard. Consult your doctor.

The problem of colic will, however, cease by the time he is four months old.

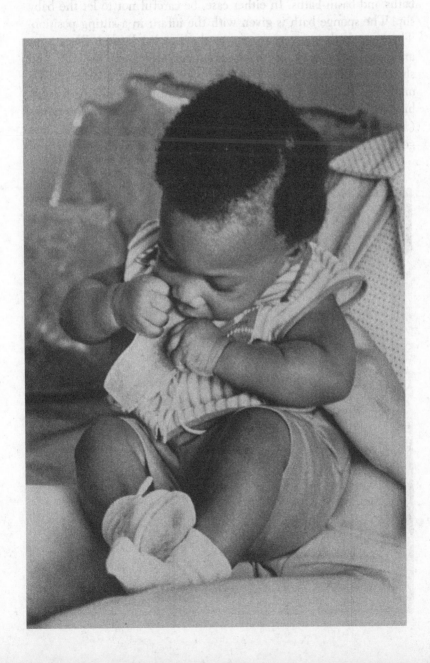

Body Care

BATHING. A regular bathing time should be established and the mood should be a happy one.

There are two types of baths you can give your infant: sponge baths and basin baths. In either case, be careful not to let the baby slip. The sponge bath is given with the infant in a sitting position. The basin bath is given as soon as the navel is healed. Place your arm across the back of the baby's neck and hold his arm and shoulder with your hand. Use a soft cloth with warm water and a mild soap. If his skin is dry, include a drop of therapeutic bath oil in his bath water. Work up a lather on the front, back, and extremities (arms, legs, feet). A new baby's skin is delicate. Handle him gently. Don't use soap on his face. Clean the outer ears and

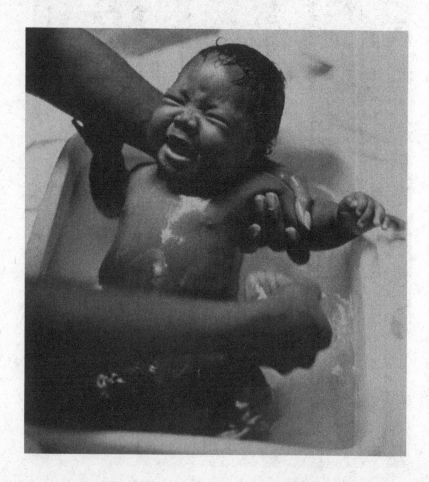

nostrils with cotton tips. Don't clean the inside of the ears where you cannot see. Make sure you dry between all his creases and folds before dressing him. Pat lotion on his body, especially if the skin is dry.

SCALP. Wash your baby's hair at least three times a week. Soap it well with a mild shampoo and rinse with a washcloth. You can hold his head in your hand with his body resting on your arm. His legs can be tucked under your arm for additional security. Brush his hair with a medium-bristled brush. If the scalp appears dry, massage it gently with petroleum jelly or an oil. There are several good hair preparations on the market to help keep infants' hair soft and manageable. Don't worry about the fontanel (soft spot), but handle it gently. Don't braid your infant's hair, especially if you have the tendency to braid tightly.

SKIN. During the first week of life, your infant's skin will begin to peel. This is normal. No special care is recommended. Within six weeks, his entire body will peel and then heal.

Don't use an excessive amount of oil on your infant's delicate skin. Many oils have been found to cause a mild rash. If your infant's skin is dry, use a dewaxed, therapeutic bath oil in his bath water.

Use petroleum jelly in the diaper area to help prevent or relieve diaper rash.

If you use a baby powder on your infant, do not shake it directly on the baby. Instead, shake the powder into your hand and then apply it to his body. This is extremely important to prevent getting powder into his lungs. In fact, put very little powder, if any at all, on your baby's chest and back.

HEAT RASH. Heat rashes are common in warm weather. Do not overdress your infant. If a heat rash develops, sponge-bath him and powder with cornstarch. Again, do not shake it directly on him.

FINGERNAILS AND TOENAILS. Keep your baby's fingernails and toenails short. Use a small pair of clean blunt-tip scissors or a nail clip. Do not file or shape your baby's nails and be careful not to cut too deeply into the cuticle. Nail care may best be handled while your baby is asleep.

EYES. The eyes may develop a secretion in the corner called "sandman's dust." Use a cotton applicator moistened with clear water to remove the secretion.

When a baby is born, silver nitrate solution is dropped into his eyes to prevent eye infection.

The average infant begins to follow light during his first week of life. He indicates awareness of his surroundings sometime during the first six weeks of life. If your infant does not show these signs by four months of age, consult a physician.

Many mothers are concerned that their infants have crossed eyes. The eye muscles take a while to develop, and the child's eyes appear to be crossed. If your infant has a broad, flat nose bridge or close-set eyes, his eyes may also appear to be crossed. This usually stabilizes by the end of his first year. If it doesn't, take him to an ophthalmologist. Crossed eyes are easily corrected.

Your child will not develop his full vision until he is about five years old. At that time, he should have 20/20 vision. You should take him to an eye specialist (ophthalmologist) before he begins school for a complete eye examination.

EARS. Clean only the outer ear or that portion of the ear that you can easily see. Do not clean the ear canals or probe into your infant's ear. Earwax is normal and helps to protect the eardrum.

Most infants develop ear infections following respiratory-tract or viral infections.

If the child has an ear infection, he will rub the ear and scream. Sometimes pus may appear. Until you are able to reach your doctor, place a heating pad or a warm towel on his ear to relieve the pain.

NOSE. Most infants experience a stuffed nose during their first year of life. Simply clean out the mucus with a cotton-tipped applicator. If the mucus is hard, moisten the applicator with water or petroleum jelly. If the nose is heavily stuffed and breathing is difficult, a vaporizer is helpful. If the condition persists, call your doctor. He may prescribe drops. Be sure to use the drops only for the exact period indicated. *Do not* give your infant nose drops before consulting your doctor.

Your infant will understand "blow your nose" before he is a year old if you repeat the phrase to him each time you want him to clean out the mucus. Teach him the correct way to blow his nose: to blow gently, one nostril at a time.

If your child should have a nosebleed, take the following steps: (1) Sit him down with head leaning slightly forward. (2) Do not allow him to blow or squeeze his nose. (3) Apply a cold towel or washcloth containing ice to the nose.

If bleeding continues or is severe, call your doctor.

MOUTH. Your baby may have a small blisterlike pucker in the center of his upper lip. This condition disappears within a few months. He may also have some tiny white pimples (epithelial "pearls") on the roof of his mouth and in the area in which the roots of his teeth are embedded. The pearls will either resorb, scale, or flake off.

TEETH. Some of your baby's teeth are formed before he is born. A small percentage of infants are born with the two lower central incisors. This is one of the reasons calcium and phosphorus are important in your diet during pregnancy and why certain drugs cannot be taken. Fluoride is important in helping to develop strong, healthy teeth and is incorporated from the mother before birth. For a time afterwards it can be given in the form of tablets, or it may be present in drinking water.

Encourage a balanced diet and proper brushing habits. A child should be taught to brush his teeth as soon as he has teeth to brush. If you have difficulty in getting him to use a toothbrush, a cotton applicator dipped in a sodium-bicarbonate solution may be used to maintain mouth hygiene during the first two years.

When your child is three, take him to see a dentist; take him earlier if you detect a dental problem before that age.

If you are not satisfied with the appearance of your child's teeth, ask a dentist about it to ease your mind or to prevent costly dental work later. Do not allow your infant to fall asleep while sucking his bottle, as this could lead to early tooth decay.

Many people believe that fevers, colds, and diarrhea are related to teething. This is not true, although teething may lower your baby's resistance and make him more prone to infections.

Teething may also cause a certain amount of discomfort and a slight rise in temperature. You can help relieve the discomfort by giving your baby a piece of hard toast, a teething ring, or baby aspirin (ask your doctor for recommended dosage), or by rubbing his gums with your clean fingers.

One important thing to remember during his teething periods is to make sure he does not chew on lead-painted objects.

The average infant begins teething around six months of age. When he reaches about two years of age, he should be the proud owner of twenty teeth. Here is an approximate timetable for teething:

Teething Chart

6 months	lower central incisors/upper central incisors
7½ months	upper lateral incisors/lower lateral incisors
10½ months	lower first molars
12½ months	upper first molars
12½ to 16½ months	upper and lower cuspids
18½ months	upper and lower second molars

If your infant's twenty teeth have not appeared by the time he is two and a half years old, you should take him to see a dentist. Dental care is not expensive. Dental neglect is.

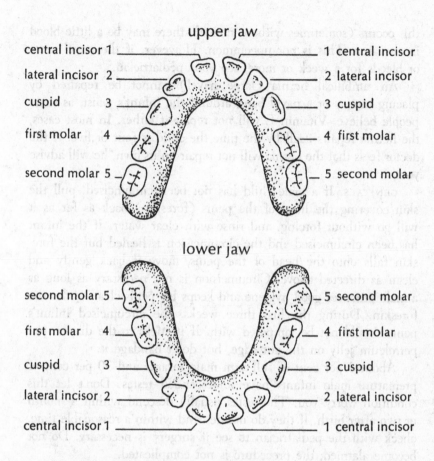

upper jaw

central incisor 1	1 central incisor
lateral incisor 2	2 lateral incisor
cuspid 3	3 cuspid
first molar 4	4 first molar
second molar 5	5 second molar

lower jaw

second molar 5	5 second molar
first molar 4	4 first molar
cuspid 3	3 cuspid
lateral incisor 2	2 lateral incisor
central incisor 1	1 central incisor

BREASTS. Swollen breasts occur in both male and female infants. If the breasts secrete a whitish substance, wipe the substance away. Do *not* squeeze the breasts. The enlargement is normal and will disappear.

NAVEL. Keep the navel clean and dry. Wash it with a mild soap, then apply some cotton dipped in a small amount of rubbing alcohol to the area. The remaining portion of the navel string usually drops off within nine days, but it can take longer. When this occurs (sometimes without notice), there may be a little blood in the area. This is not uncommon. However, if the navel spots or bleeds for a week or more, see your pediatrician.

An umbilical hernia (large navel) cannot be repaired by placing money or a navel band around the infant's waist, as some people believe. Vitamin E will not repair it either. In most cases, the hernia repairs itself by the time the child is four or five. If the doctor feels that the hernia will not repair on its own, he will advise you.

GENITALS. If a male child has not been circumcised, pull the skin covering the head of the penis (foreskin) back as far as it will go without forcing, and rinse with clear water. If the infant has been circumcised and the circumcision is healed but the foreskin falls onto the head of the penis, move it back gently and clean as directed above. Circumcision is not necessary as long as a male practices good hygiene and keeps his penis clean under the foreskin. During the first three weeks, the circumcised infant's penis should not be tampered with. If it sticks to the diaper, put petroleum jelly on the cut edge, but don't bandage it.

About 3 per cent of full-term male infants and 30 per cent of premature male infants have undescended testes. Don't let this condition worry you. The testes usually descend within a month or two after birth. If they do not descend within a reasonable time, check with the pediatrician to see if surgery is necessary. Do not become alarmed; the procedure is not complicated.

In a female infant, use a cotton applicator moistened with clear water to clean gently between the folds of the vulva (vaginal lips) in a downward motion—from front to back. A little blood and whitish discharge during the first few days should not alarm you. This is common. Many people call it the "first menstrual flow."

Always clean around the mouth of the vagina and check to see if there is an opening. Many female infants' vaginal mouths will close during the first weeks of life without the mother's knowledge since some women are fearful of hurting the baby and do not always clean the area.

DIAPERS. Your infant should be changed before and after each feeding and immediately after a bowel movement. Keeping him dry will help prevent diaper rash. It is not necessary to wake your infant to change him simply because he is wet. If he is uncomfortable, he will let you know.

When changing diapers, be sure to clean the genital areas with warm water, as directed earlier. If the baby has had a bowel movement, clean away all of the feces before washing. Remember to clean the penis or vagina. Dry the baby thoroughly and massage the genital area and buttocks with petroleum jelly. A powder is not necessary. Do not pin the diapers to the undershirt.

Clothing

The most important article in your baby's wardrobe is a stack of diapers—no less than three dozen. Your baby does not care whether they are cloth or disposable so long as he is dry and comfortable.

He will need at least three nightgowns and four undershirts, a receiving blanket, and a heavier blanket. Rubber pants may be worn to keep down wetness.

Always keep his feet covered; they are the hardest to keep warm.

The simple rule in infant dress is: keep him dry, clean, and suitably dressed for the weather.

DIAPER CARE. If you decide to use washable diapers, wash them daily. Soiled diapers should be rinsed first in the toilet bowl. Never put soiled diapers in a pan to soak before rinsing them thoroughly. Use a rust-proof covered pail to store the diapers until you are ready to wash them. Always keep the water level equal to the level of the diapers. If you wish, you may add a mild laundry detergent to the water while they are soaking.

CLOTHING CARE. It is a good practice to wash all of your baby's soiled clothes at the same time, diapers in one batch and the rest of the clothing in another. Use hot water and a mild detergent. You may also add a teaspoon of bicarbonate of soda to laundry water. Rinse thoroughly. Do not wash your infant's clothing with the family laundry, to avoid bacterial contamination.

Rest

Each baby is different in temperament and mood. You cannot always set up a four-hour sleeping schedule, but you can make his rest periods quiet and comfortable. There is no need to keep the house absolutely quiet because the baby is sleeping.

Your baby should have his own sleeping area and bed. The sleeping equipment should be comfortable and safe. Make sure that the crib has sidings and that the bars are not so far apart that his head will go through. Place bumpers around the sides. This is just another precautionary measure. The mattress should be firm. A pillow is not advisable. Keep the mattress covered with a waterproof fabric, but never allow the infant to lie directly on rubber or plastic. Never use a dry-cleaning bag or any thin plastic to cover your baby's mattress. Hang bright articles over the crib and on the sides for his amusement.

Most babies enjoy sleeping on their stomachs. This is a good practice, especially when they are very young and unable to turn over if they spit up milk or mucus.

Development

In the beginning, your infant will be unable to hold his head up. When handling him you must always support his head. During his first week of life, he will lie on his back with his head facing in the direction you place it. Most babies keep one arm outstretched and the other next to their heads or chests.

104   *Infant and Child Care*

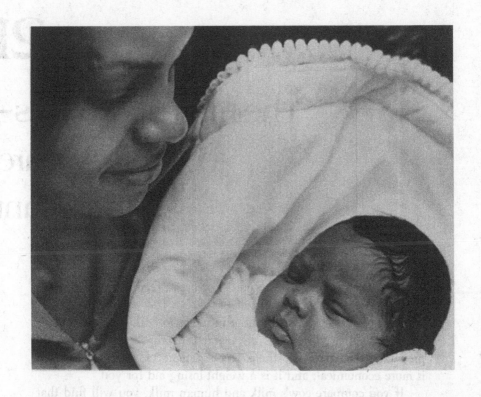

Before the end of the first week, your infant may be able to turn his head, follow an object or light, and watch you while you feed him or talk. By the end of his first six weeks, he may be able to raise himself a few inches while holding his head up. He may also show enthusiasm when you take out your breast or show him his bottle at feeding time. He begins to coo and laugh aloud. He may also smile when you smile at him. By the end of six weeks he may be able to hold his head erect if his body is supported. He may put his hands together and watch them in play, or reach for objects. Never leave him unattended on the changing table or a bed. He may just flip over.

You will find your new baby eager to learn and fun to watch.

21

The First Six Weeks–
Dietary Care
of the Infant

FEEDING. The decision to bottle- or breast-feed is a personal one and you should make it yourself.

Breast-feeding offers several advantages to both the new mother and the infant: the milk is always at the proper temperature; no preparation is involved; there is no danger of contamination; it is more economical; and it is a weight-losing aid for you.

If you compare cow's milk and human milk, you will find that cow's milk contains a higher percentage of protein. However, this is the least digestible part of cow's milk and the part that forms curds. Human milk contains more sugar. The fat content of the two milks is about the same. Although most infants have no difficulty digesting the fat of cow's milk, the type of fat present in human milk is more easily digestible.

Cow's milk and human milk have equal calorie contents— twenty calories per ounce. The mineral content of cow's milk is higher. However, neither cow's milk nor human milk contains adequate amounts of iron. The baby compensates for this by using the iron supply stored away while in his mother's womb. This supply lasts approximately four months. In a premature infant, iron stores are not as plentiful, and iron supplements usually have to be given.

Human milk contains more vitamin C, while cow's milk contains more riboflavin and thiamine. Both milks have small amounts of vitamin D and large quantities of vitamin A. The content of water is the same in both.

Some infants may require a special formula if they are allergic to cow's milk or have lactose deficiency. These infants are usually fed soybean milk or goat's milk.

BREAST-FEEDING. If you have decided to breast-feed your infant, you should note that milk is not secreted until six to twelve hours after delivery. Meanwhile you will secrete a thick, yellowish liquid called colostrum, which is highly beneficial to your infant, since it contains antibodies that can help protect him from many diseases and viral infections during the first six months of his life. While this natural immunity is extremely valuable, it is not a substitute for the immunizations that should be started, regardless of diet, at about two months of age.

The first two or three feedings should be brief—two to three minutes—to avoid cracking of the nipples. Thereafter the baby should be fed for about ten minutes on each side every four hours. Of course, some babies may need more frequent feedings, some less frequent. The breasts should be alternated at each feeding, and, if possible, emptied each time.

If you have a premature or low-birth-weight infant, you may still be able to feed him breast milk if you extract it with your hands or with a breast pump and store it in a bottle. Discuss this with your doctor.

You can feed your baby either lying down or sitting up. If you decide to sit while feeding him, lean forward, holding the infant with one arm and allowing him to rest on your lap. Be sure to hold the breast away from the infant's nose so that he can breathe. It is important that you and your baby are comfortable. You should also talk to him and caress him gently while feeding to add to his sense of security.

You need not put any special ointments on your nipples to disinfect them, and do not use boric acid. Nature keeps them healthy if you keep your body and clothing clean. Simply wash them with warm water before and after each feeding.

Some babies refuse to feed during the first few days. If your infant doesn't want to eat, don't force him. Continue to hold him next to your breast until he is ready. Eventually, he will come around.

A common complaint in breast-feeding is cracked or sore nipples. If a baby continues to suck at a nipple from which no milk is flowing, nipples will often crack or become sore.

In that event, keep the nipples dry and exposed to air when you are not feeding to help heal them. Be sure to tell your doctor about the soreness, especially if it is accompanied with fever. He may prescribe medication to help arrest the soreness. While you are breast-feeding, *do not* take any medication, including aspirin, before consulting your doctor.

It is not uncommon for a sore or cracked nipple to bleed. The small amount of blood that may get into the baby's mouth is harmless.

Women often say that they didn't breast-feed their children because they didn't have enough milk. This problem is more imagined than real. The size of your breasts has no relationship to the amount of milk you produce. Most women have an adequate quantity and quality of milk if the baby sleeps for about four hours between feedings and gains weight normally. Anxiety and concern, however, may often decrease the milk flow.

You will require additional foods to compensate for those calories secreted in your milk and for those required for milk production. Your diet should be high in vitamins, proteins, fluids, and minerals. Certain foods that you eat may cause stomach discomfort or loose stools in the nursing infant. They include cabbage, onions, tomatoes, and chocolate. Watch your infant for reactions, and if no problems arise, you may safely eat these foods.

Certain other substances transmitted from the mother to the baby can occasionally be harmful. The most common are medications such as atropine, the barbiturates, and some antibiotics.

Cigarette smoking is *forbidden* for the nursing mother because the nicotine gets into the milk. If this should occur, the infant may have difficulty gaining weight. It has also been found that infants who breathe smoke during the first year of life are more likely to suffer serious lung and respiratory disorders that could lead to permanent damage.

Your milk supply varies during the first few months. If your breasts begin to leak, pad your bra, press your nipples, or try to get your infant on a rigid feeding schedule. If your milk supply is lower at the end of the day, relax, it will replenish itself within a short period of time. If your milk supply does not come back to its original level, you may try nursing more often or emptying your breasts with a pump or by hand, to help restore your supply. Rest is also beneficial.

Engorgement is an abnormal fullness or distension of the breasts. Some fullness, of course, is normal at the onset of the nursing period, but if it progresses to pain and stoppage of milk flow, consult your doctor.

Infections of the breast may necessitate discontinuance of nursing. Typhoid fever, infectious hepatitis, active tuberculosis, and malaria require that you cease breast-feeding your infant immediately. A mother with severe mental disorders and deficient nutrition should not breast-feed either.

Weaning from the breast can be done at any age. A mother who goes back to work can substitute formula for one or two feedings. Cereals can usually be started around two months of age, fruits and vegetables at three months, and meats at five months of age. In some cultures women wean their infants as soon as they

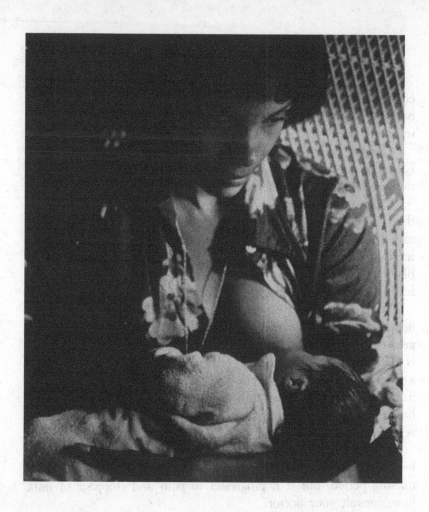

are pregnant again because they believe that breast milk becomes poisonous. There is no truth in this.

If you must wean your infant from your breast before he is six months of age, wean him to a formula, using cow's or goat's milk, whichever your doctor prescribes.

A working mother can continue to provide her infant with her own milk during the day by storing milk pumped from her breast in a sterilized container. She can also do this to help keep up her supply of milk. When she is not at work, she can nurse the infant as usual.

Breast-feeding is important for you and your infant. It may take a month or two before you and your baby reach a happy medium at feeding time. This is not uncommon. Be patient! Eat a well-balanced diet, drink plenty of fluids, and get a lot of rest. And enjoy it!

FORMULA-FEEDING. There are two types of formula-feedings available today. The first is a ready-mixed formula, which may require the addition of sterilized water, given to the baby with no further preparation. The second type has to be mixed. There is no basic difference between them. Both provide good nutrition. It is estimated that 80 per cent of infants in the United States are formula-fed.

Here is how to prepare a formula at home if you choose to follow this method.

All the utensils must be washed in hot water and detergent and then rinsed in hot water. The bottles and nipples must be sterilized. The formula consists of thirteen ounces of evaporated milk, nineteen ounces of water, and two tablespoons of white corn syrup. This mixture is poured into sterilized formula bottles. Four ounces in each bottle (eight bottles) will suffice in the early weeks. The sterilized nipples are now placed upside down on the bottles (leave rings or caps closed). Place the bottles inside a wire rack or on a towel in a deep pan filled with three inches of water. (Use a sterilizer if one is available.) Bring the water to a boil, cover the pot, and boil for another twenty-five minutes. Make sure the pan is cool before removing the bottles. Screw the caps on the bottles tightly and place them in the refrigerator.

At feeding time take a bottle from the refrigerator, invert the nipple, and warm it to room temperature by placing it in a pan of hot water. Test the temperature by squirting a few drops of formula on your wrist. The nipple holes should be just large enough to let the milk go through slowly.

The room in which you feed your baby should be quiet and free from distractions, and you should be relaxed. Hold the baby in your lap with his head well-supported, raised slightly, and resting at an angle. Keep him close to your body and talk to him as you would if you were breast-feeding. No air should get into the nipple area. This is accomplished by always keeping the nipple end full of milk. The baby should be burped once during feeding and again after feeding.

To burp your infant, place a clean towel or clean diaper on your shoulder. Hold the baby over your shoulder for a few minutes, patting him gently on the back. The purpose of burping your infant is to bring up the air swallowed during feeding. This helps avoid abdominal discomfort. Many babies spit up a small amount of milk after feeding. This is normal.

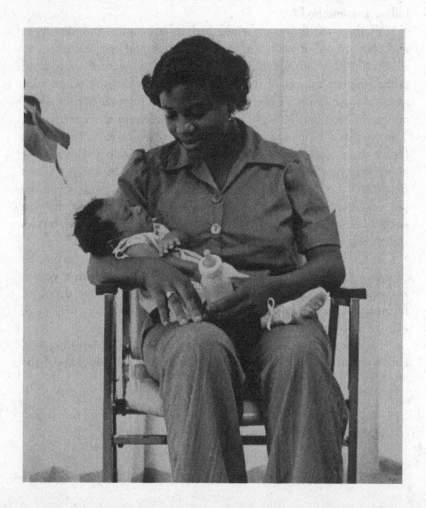

22

Your Child – Six Weeks to Four Months

The first six weeks of your child's life will be trying for you, especially if this is your first child.

At the end of that time your infant has probably made great advances. His features are now more clearly defined, and you may be able to tell whether he looks like you, his father, or his grandparents. He has probably gained about two or three pounds. If he hasn't been able to roll over from his back to his side before the end of the sixth week, he will probably do so now. Watch him. By this time he will already have begun to recognize you and your voice, to discover his own voice, to play in his bath, and to stay awake just a little bit longer.

By the time he is four months old, he has more than likely gained about three pounds and grown about three inches. He may be able to sit up without support, turn over from his back, notice other people and objects, and move about on his stomach. Some infants are also able to crawl on their knees or move backward; some move forward using only one leg to do the pushing.

Your infant is a social being: he will smile when you smile and laugh when you laugh. You will not need to tickle him to get this response. He will want to be held more often or wish to sit un-supported. In essence, he is capable of making his desires known.

Most black infants during this period enjoy play and music. You should provide both. Whatever music you select, keep the volume at a comfortable level. Music played too loud might affect his hearing.

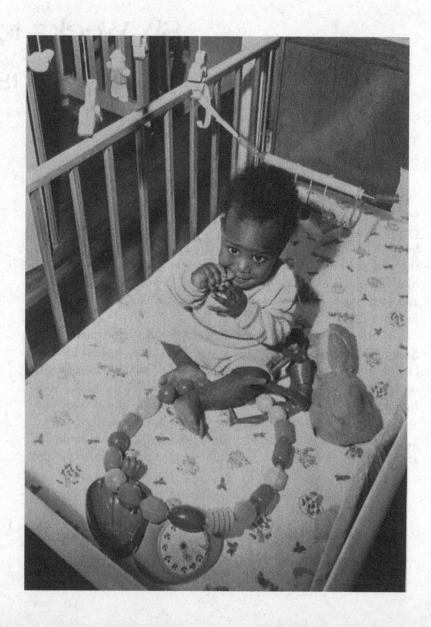

Clear an area for play, put down a blanket, bedspread, or sheet, remove dangerous objects and let him loose. He is now ready for small soft toys, especially a bright-colored ball that he can follow. A playpen is best if there are other children playing nearby, or if there are animals. Place a heavy chair or hassock next to the play area so that he will have something to pull himself up on.

Between three and four months, he will begin to sit up. A chair swing or jump-up swing are good exercise, as they help strengthen leg muscles, and they are fun, too.

Your baby observes everything, including the television. He will have no problem handling his rattle or holding his teething ring. If he is using a bottle, he may prefer holding it himself. Allow him to do so, but watch him closely because he may become bored and drop it.

He must have his first checkup at six weeks. If this is the season of upper respiratory infections, ask your doctor to examine carefully for any possible disorders of this kind. If you've neglected to take him in for a six weeks' checkup, do not neglect to take him in at two months for his diphtheria, whooping cough (pertussis), and tetanus injection (see page 163). You will have to return six weeks later for a second D.P.T. immunization. The doctor will also administer the poliomyelitis antigen by mouth. It has a sweet taste and the infant will like it. At four months, he gets the second dose of the antigen. You will be given a record of immunizations. Keep it. Your child will need it when he enters school, travels, or does anything requiring such information.

During this period you should continue to feed your infant sterilized formula, although you may now add small amounts of cereal to it. Larger amounts of cereal may be given gradually, depending upon his appetite.

Even though he may wish to hold his own bottle, you should continue to hold him close to your breast. He still needs to feel that he is loved.

Your baby's hair is now changing to its natural state. You may help to keep it soft and manageable by using some of the new hair products, such as "hair food," normally found in the black community and recommended for infants. The hair should be kept clean, brushed, and moderately oiled.

Bathing your infant is a lot of fun provided you don't mind getting wet. He will enjoy splashing and kicking. You must continue to hold him securely: a lot of movement in that small baby tub may turn it over.

Many infants are very strong. Hold your baby carefully. He may try to jump out of your arms.

Don't allow him to cry until he is exhausted simply because you are trying to prevent him from becoming spoiled. You don't spoil a child by taking care of his needs and giving him love.

23

Your Child— Four Months to Six Months

You will now probably spend a lot of time chasing your baby. He, in turn, is spending most of his waking hours testing his skills, moving about independently. The average black infant starts crawling between four and six months of age. Some crawl before and some wait until they are eight or nine months old. But even if your child does not crawl before nine months of age you shouldn't worry. He will get around to it. Try not to be overprotective. Give him the space and freedom to move about. His inability to crawl now does not mean that he is mentally retarded. He is probably just cautious.

If you leave him alone to play, you will hear him laughing and squealing. He will be enjoying himself and listening to his voice. If you encourage him with praise, he will continue to use his newly found ability.

Don't be alarmed when he objects to your taking something away from him, or out of his sight. If he has already begun to move about independently, he may try to recover the item himself. Many infants learn cute tricks. They may cough or clear their throats or bang on objects to hear the noise. At this stage your infant may also sit in his own chair; say "da-da"; get his first tooth; stand while being held or by holding onto a chair or play-pen; hold larger objects; notice every tiny speck on the floor; pick up things and put them into his mouth; transfer objects from one hand to another; and sit for longer periods without wishing to be disturbed. As long as he's not hurting himself, don't interfere. Let him move at his own pace.

Your baby might try to imitate your speech and movement. If you bang on the table, he may bang on the table. If you make certain simple sounds, he may attempt to make the same sounds. He will try many new moves. If he is unable to master them, he may become very angry.

Allison was a determined infant. The day she was three months old, she was lying on her play blanket, enjoying herself. Suddenly

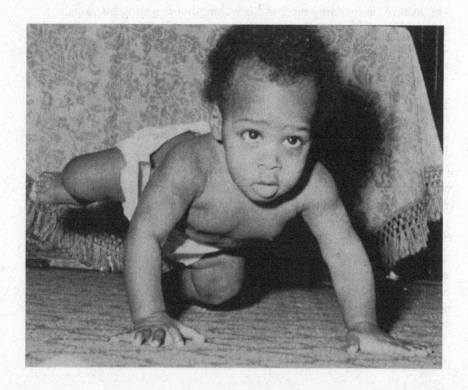

she flipped over from her stomach to her back and then from her back to her stomach. She wanted to do it again. But to no avail. She became frustrated and cried herself to sleep. When she awoke several hours later, she tried again until she finally flipped from her back to her stomach several times with ease.

Infants like Allison do not give up easily. They will continue to have that type of determination throughout their lives if properly motivated. When you see your child trying to reach a goal, even at this very young age, encourage him, applaud him, give him a kiss.

When your infant is six months, you no longer need to sterilize bottles. You must, however, continue to keep his bottles and nipples as clean as possible. Use a cap to cover the nipple while not in use. Give him regular milk.

If your doctor decides that this is the best time to start him on solid foods, you need not purchase prepared foods. It is much more economical to get a blender or a simple food mill and grind down your infant's food. It is tastier, more nutritional, and contains no additives. Introduce solid foods to your infant one at a time. In case he is allergic to one, you will be able to know which one caused the allergy. Don't give your child pork or beef at this time. Feed him egg yolks, cheese, and other protein-providing foods.

Blended canned fruits can also be fed to the infant who is six months or older.

Your baby's appetite may decrease when you change his diet to more food and less milk. Don't force him to eat. Give him a cup for his milk. This may teach him how to use a cup and help wean him as well. Also use the cup for other drinks. Some parents enjoy giving their infants a little beer. However, doctors often advise against giving orange juice until children are older, since many are allergic to it. Discuss this with your physician.

The new diet may cause a change in your child's bowel habits and the consistency and color of his stool. So don't be alarmed if you see a red stool. You probably fed him beets.

If your doctor recommended vitamins for your infant before you left the hospital, you should continue to use them. Do not add supplementary doses of vitamins such as A, D, or E to those you already have. The amounts of vitamins and iron recommended for your child at birth are adequate unless otherwise advised by your physician.

While your infant is getting teeth, he may drool a lot and be irritable. He may also have a slight temperature. Don't panic. Check his gums to see if the bottom middle teeth are trying to protrude. If he is teething, he will need a little more attention. Give him teething rings and one-half of a baby aspirin or Tylenol.

At six months take your infant to the pediatrician or clinic for his third poliomyelitis shot. This is essential.

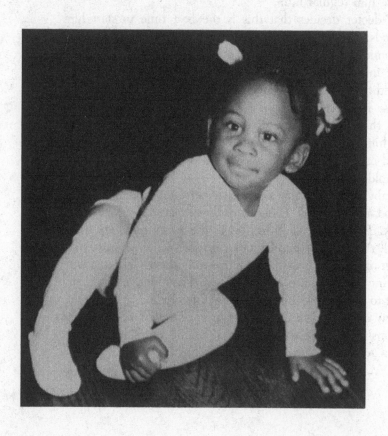

He should by now have doubled his birth weight and grown about six inches. If he was born with dark blue or red spots the dark ones may still be present. Normally they disappear by the time the child is four. Your child's body, including his arms and legs, may be a shade darker than his face. This, too, evens out by the time he is four. If his eyes don't focus properly, take him to your physician or the eye specialist at the clinic. Also make sure that your child's legs and feet are forming properly. If he is bowlegged or his toes turn in or out severely, report it to your doctor. Such problems can be corrected if caught in time.

24

Your Child–
Six Months to
Twelve Months

This is a very active period for you and your infant. Put up the guard at the top of the steps and a screen in front of your fireplace; lock away medicines and poisonous cleaning materials; clear your floor of dangerous articles such as pins and needles; clear away plaster and lead-painted objects. Your infant is on his way.

He is curious, explorative, demanding, and eager to learn. Talk to him; "read" to him by pointing out objects in picture books; love him and enjoy him.

Some infants develop faster, some slower. We are using the average motor-development pattern for black infants. Between six to twelve months, your infant will grow another three or four inches and gain another five or six pounds. His skin will normally be clear unless he has a rash or "liver spots," and his hair will have reached its natural state. It is sometimes helpful to wet and oil your child's hair before brushing it. Treat it gently. Don't make your child unhappy because of the texture of his hair. Hair texture is inherited. Hair care is your responsibility.

The average infant now begins to recognize familiar people and objects. This is the time to show him a few cards with pictures and captions of a house, dog, cat, horse, and so on. You can easily make your own. For the "mommy" and "daddy" cards, paste photographs of you and his father over the picture already on the card. You can make cards for the other members of the family as well. For the animal cards, imitate the animal sounds. He will probably have no problem imitating sounds and motions, and he may be able to tell from the tone of your voice and your actions what you are trying to tell him. He wants to learn to speak. Talk to him slowly, using short sentences and, where possible, pointing out the objects as you say them. He is ready to communicate now and needs your guidance and patience. By the time he is one, he will understand much of what you say, even though he may not be able to say it himself. Keep on talking to help develop his speech and vocabulary. Try to avoid "un, huh," "un, un" and "huh?" You want your child to learn to speak, not grunt.

During this period, your infant may also discover his genitals and will find much pleasure playing with them. Don't discourage him. He is exploring his body. You may help him by naming the parts of his body, using the correct terms, such as penis.

Your infant may begin to sleep for longer periods during the night, and he may experience dreams or nightmares and wake up often. In many cases, he is simply suffering the pain of teething. Whatever the case, do not make a habit of taking him to bed with you to comfort him. If he cries, go to his bed, speak to him softly, and help him go back to sleep. If he is teething, one-half of a baby aspirin or Tylenol may be helpful. Give him a glass of water but avoid giving him a bottle because he may fall asleep with the bottle in his mouth.

At this age you may wean your baby from breast-feeding to a bottle. Of course, some mothers have been very successful in weaning their infants directly to a cup or a glass. (You can decrease your breast-milk supply by cutting back on your baby's sucking and your fluid intake.) Whether you wean your baby to a bottle or cup, it takes time and patience.

Your infant should get his third D.P.T. at this age. By the time he is one he must be given the measles, mumps, and rubella vaccine and be tested for TB.

Your infant may begin to pull himself up to a standing position between six and nine months of age. Remove dangerous objects such as scissors, knives, china, and glassware from the tables. Don't use a tablecloth because he may pull it off and whatever else is on the table with it.

Your infant may be able to climb stairs by the time he is nine months old or whenever he begins to crawl. However, he may not learn to go down the steps until about three months later, so leave up the guard rail.

At the age of seven months your child may be able to take his first step by holding on to an object and will probably take his first step alone by the time he is ten months. Within another two weeks the black child may be able to walk alone with ease and coordination.

Well before this period, he should recognize a musical beat. By the time he is a year old, he may try to imitate you or performers he has seen on television.

When your infant is a year old, he should have about six teeth. You no longer need to blend his food, but it must still be chopped fine. If he is used to table foods, he will not accept commercially prepared chopped foods. He will now be getting four additional teeth. Give him bones to gnaw on for taste and teething comfort. Most infants enjoy steak and pork-chop bones. See that your child continues to get well-balanced meals. You do not want to hinder his ability to explore and learn because of a poor diet.

The average ten-month-old black infant may be a little shy but he will probably be able to wave and say "bye-bye"; raise his finger to say he is one year old; call "mama" and "daddy"; participate and try to lead in "pat-a-cake" and other nursery games; understand and follow certain orders, such as "Get me a clean diaper"; and make marks on paper.

TOILET TRAINING. Many parents are able to toilet train their infants during this period. There is no specific age at which to start as long as the training is one of pleasure and not one of torment and stress.

On the morning that Lisa was thirteen months old, she went into the kitchen where her mother was washing dishes and said, "Mommy, boo boo." Her mother looked at her and nodded. Lisa again said, "Mommy, boo boo," while pulling off her pants. The mother quickly got the message and took her to the toilet.

Lisa's mother was surprised that her child was ready to be toilet trained. She realized that whenever Lisa soiled her diapers she had used the term "boo boo." Lisa associated "boo boo" with her bowel movement and was therefore easy to train at home. However, Lisa was not toilet trained when away from home or away from her mother until she was eighteen months old.

Learning to use the toilet can be a marvelous experience for both mother and child. A child enjoys pleasing and the mother enjoys the freedom of not having to clean soiled diapers.

Many black mothers must return to work early in their child's life and are impatient with toilet training. If your child has made rapid progress in his first stages of life, he will probably do so when the time comes to toilet train him. Give him the same kind of encouragement that you gave him when he began to crawl and walk.

To toilet train your child, you must observe him closely, even before he is one year of age. He will give signs when he is about to have a bowel movement. He may bend over, pull at his pants, turn red in the face, or grunt. Take him to the pot to sit. Use either a small training pot or a training seat that fits on a regular toilet. If you use the latter, place a footstool under his feet to make him comfortable and secure. Do not make him sit too long. It will help if you stay with him. Praise him when he is finished.

Always respond when he asks to go to the bathroom. Never say, "We are not at home," or "You have on a diaper, use it." This only confuses the infant and slows down his training.

Although urine training takes a little bit longer, most black infants are daytime toilet trained (urine and bowel movement) between two and two and a half years of age. They may still need you, however, to help them take down their underwear and put it back on.

While you are toilet training your child, you must also train him in hygiene. Give him paper and show him how to wipe himself. Teach your child to wipe away from his genitals. This is particularly important for the female. Many vaginal infections are caused by poor toilet habits. Your child may not learn how to clean himself properly until he is three or four years old, so please be patient.

When he is finished, show him how to wash his hands with soap and water and then dry them thoroughly. Good hygiene begins early. Do not make a big issue of these things if the child forgets or has an accident. Once you begin to apply too much pressure and show signs of anxiety, you make toilet hygiene difficult.

Teaching a boy to stand while urinating takes a little longer than training a girl to sit while she urinates. Perhaps his father, a big brother, or another male would be the best teacher for this, since young children like to imitate.

The average child is able to stay dry during the night by the time he is two and a half years old. However, night training may not be completed before he is three or more. You may help by encouraging him to empty his bladder before going to sleep. If a child does experience difficulty in staying dry during the night, do not tease or scold him. Most of all, do not withhold water from him when he is thirsty. Withholding fluid intake can cause dehydration.

When your child is about one, he may have a temper tantrum, especially if he is unable to get a mission accomplished. Don't allow it to upset you. See what is causing the problem. If a toy is stuck somewhere, show him how to release it. Then tell him that the tantrum didn't help, his effort did. If you continue to show him how to handle situations rather than suffer frustrations, his temper tantrums will soon end.

The average black infant is capable of learning and understanding before he is twelve months old. He is also able to follow simple instructions, and perhaps make simple judgments.

Although many child specialists have said that the infant's motor development has nothing to do with his intelligence, this is not true.

Diana was seven months of age when her mother agreed to have her participate in a university infant test designed to determine if younger crawling infants could see as well as older crawling infants. Diana was placed on a large table, along with other infants. There were red and white squares on the surface of one-half of the table. The squares continued on the other half of the table, which was depressed about twelve inches. The entire table was covered with a heavy glass. One half of the table was obviously safe. The other half of the table *looked* unsafe since the squares were a foot deep. The examiner placed the babies on the obviously safe side and the mothers at the other end. The mothers were asked to plead with their children to come to them, using smiles or whatever method of encouragement they felt would work.

All of the infants crawled toward their mothers until they reached the center of the table where the squares gave an unsafe illusion. They began to cry but their mothers continued to call them. All of them refused to move. Finally, after much consideration and many tears, Diana reached out toward the other end of the table to test its durability and proceeded to crawl only as far as she had tested. Crying all the way, she tested the entire distance in this manner until she had reached her mother, where she again felt safe. .

The examiners said that Diana crawled to her mother because she did not have the ability of the other infants to recognize the illusion. Did Diana really crawl to her mother because she could not see as well, or was she using her young mind to analyze and make a decision regarding the situation? Even though Diana trusted her mother, she did not proceed until she herself was sure the area was safe. Was this a sign of intelligence or a motor-development skill?

This example is given because many child specialists have concluded that even though the average black infant has an accelerated gross motor development, this has no bearing on his intelligence. Diana's case is an example of how the system refuses to recognize certain obvious intellectual points regarding blacks. Normally, if they admit to something this obvious, they usually say that it is a "unique" situation.

As a black parent, you must be aware of this type of degradation and protect your child from it. The same type of rationale used in the interpretation of this test may be used to evaluate the performance of your child under varying circumstances.

25

Your Child–
Twelve Months to
Eighteen Months

Now that your infant is a year old, he will be more independent and more active. It will be very difficult to keep him in a restricted area or a playpen unless you provide him with blocks and boxes to work with. Even that diversion will not last long. The bold toddler now enjoys being chased and may pause just long enough to give you the opportunity to catch him. He likes to play with everything, so long as you are nearby. While you are in the kitchen, he may want to help you. Give him a lower drawer or cabinet that he can call his own and use as he pleases. He enjoys peek-a-boo and pat-a-cake more now that he can initiate the play.

Be careful what you put in your wastebaskets, on lower bookshelves, and in lower drawers. He is an explorer every inch of the way. He knows each room in your house or apartment and will not hesitate to get what he wants without your help.

You may now have help in dressing your infant. He will hold his arms up for you to put on his shirt and lift his feet when he sees the slacks coming. Undressing is more fun and he will probably do it without your help.

Bathing is a pleasure for the one-year-old. He will enjoy playing in the tub. Let him wash himself but don't leave him alone in the bathroom.

Identifying the parts of his body is a lot of fun for him. He will name the eyes, nose, mouth, teeth, and so on, not only on you and himself but also on his toy animals and the people on the television screen. Cheer him for his accomplishments.

Books are even more enjoyable now because he can turn the pages and identify some of the pictures. He may also try to throw a ball (unsuccessfully), and he will insist upon holding his spoon while you feed him. He will also enjoy turning the lights on and off.

Most children will be a "babies" to him now and he will happily point them out to you wherever he is.

Play activities should be chosen to fit a baby's learning range. Some infants between twelve and eighteen months enjoy swings and swimming. Try to make physical activities available to him. His muscles as well as his mind need building up.

Your baby will know how to protest now, either by gestures or by a simple "no." He will enjoy throwing things and watching them fall, even when not protesting. Dropping things is even more fun if you are around to pick them up. Don't let this upset you, for it will pass as he continues to develop.

Until your child is five, he should wear shoes only when he goes outdoors. In the house, he can go around without shoes so he can exercise his foot muscles. However, be sure to keep your floor clean and free of dangerous objects. Being barefoot allows the child to develop agility and strength. It also toughens the bottoms of his feet. If you insist upon having your child's feet covered at home, let him wear slippers, socks, or thongs. When you buy shoes make sure they are roomy and flexible through the arch. Allow his feet to grow naturally, without restriction. There should be about three-fourths of an inch between the end of the toe and the end of the shoe. Also, be sure that the shoes are wide enough.

Provide your child with stimulating toys and playmates. He

will like both. He may not exactly play with the friend, but he will enjoy his company so long as there is no biting, snatching, or pushing. Your child should have a playmate of his own age or an older one (three or four years older) who enjoys teaching him.

If your baby has watched you brush your teeth, he may insist on brushing his own. Let him. He will not be able to do it properly, but he will develop a valuable habit.

Your child is ready for more discipline now. This does not necessarily mean spanking, however. He will challenge you and want to do things his way, such as refusing to nap, having a temper tantrum, or examining a light socket or plug. This is the time for guiding discipline. Tell him that he must take his afternoon nap; that he must learn to handle problems rather than scream; that he must not examine light sockets. Be *firm* and *consistent*. That is the only way to achieve sound discipline.

The first poliomyelitis booster shot is due between fifteen and eighteen months of age. Attend to it promptly. If you are planning to travel abroad, your infant should have a smallpox vaccination. This immunization is no longer needed in the United States because the incidence of smallpox is very low.

Most children's appetites diminish during this period and many like to feed themselves. Give your child foods that he can pick up with his fingers and let him feed himself if he insists. It may be messy but it's good for him. If he doesn't eat everything that you place before him, don't panic. Above all, don't ever force your child to eat. Overweight babies become overweight adults and are prime candidates for hypertension and heart disease. I am sure you have often heard people comment with pleasure about how fat the baby is. This type of flattery encourages the parents to harass the youngsters into overeating: "Boy, eat this food before I stuff it down your throat," or, "Eat all of your food and grow to be big and strong." Your baby will grow big and strong without your fussing or conning. Let him eat as much or as little as he wants. Don't make an issue of eating.

The eighteen-month-old infant will continue to make rapid progress. He will say more words, act more independently, and enjoy a greater variety of experiences. He will imitate almost everything you do. Give him love and sound guidance. Give him freedom to learn and the courage to continue. His ability to become a self-respecting adult is developing.

26

Your Child–
Eighteen Months
to Two Years

Eighteen months to two years is a great learning period. Your child is eager to do things. He is also eager and ready to communicate. He will want to feed himself, and will tell you when he is ready to eat. When you are setting the table, he will know that the rest of the family should be called to dinner: "Daddy, eat," he will say in no uncertain terms. "Sit down." He may now begin to test his potential by pushing, biting, hitting, or taking things from smaller children. He may even bite you. The eighteen-month-old infant is possessive and may not enjoy sharing. If he sees you sitting in his chair, he may ask you to move.

Your infant might now show a keen sense of observation. For example, Cheryl awoke to find that her mother had moved the sofa and chairs to another area of the living room. As soon as she walked into the room she started touching the moved articles and commenting on the change in her own little way: "Oh, oh. Oh, oh."

If something spills, he may grab the mop or a rag and clean it up. He may also be ready to keep his diapers dry, so with gentle encouragement you may be able to get him to tell you when he has to urinate or have a bowel movement. He may also learn to clean himself after a bowel movement and flush the toilet.

There isn't very much that your beautiful black infant will miss when you take him for a walk. You need patience. He will walk slowly and examine and question everything along the way. Don't discourage this inquisitiveness. Answer his questions and point out extra things for him.

You should now have no problem in getting him to help you save steps. Ask him and he will gladly get a clean diaper, put paper in the wastebasket, wash and dry his hands, and do other helpful things.

During this period, he will also repeat portions of verses, parts of the alphabet, and numbers.

Learning is fun for your child. He loves to look at books and identify the objects for you. Don't forget to let him know how pleased you are with him.

If you have taken your infant to a roadside restaurant once, you won't be able to pass one ever again without his asking for French fries.

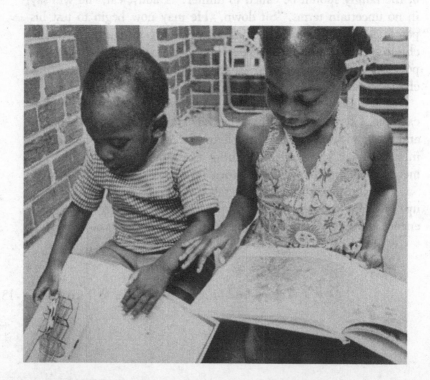

Telephone conversations are fun during this period, and he will want to be in on most of your conversations. If you have friends who don't mind talking to a toddler, let him talk. You may want to get him a toy telephone to use for his make-believe conversations while you are using yours.

Television programs such as *Sesame Street* are educational and enjoyable for his young mind. They help him to learn his alphabet and count, and also teach him to think. Include *Sesame Street* in your child's daily schedule. It will keep him occupied while he picks up quite a bit of information. Once he sees this show, he may insist on watching it regularly. However, too much television is not advised, since it does not provide children with the guided active learning—for example, reading and writing—that only you or another teacher can provide.

There are a number of excellent educational toys available, such as magnetic letters (they can be placed on the refrigerator and other metal surfaces), odd-shaped blocks, coloring books and crayons, and nursery-song records. Try to provide some of these teaching aids for your youngster.

You will now have to watch your shoes and purses. For your child enjoys imitating now more than ever. He will be trying on shoes of all sizes and shapes and trundling back and forth. He may stuff your purse with blocks and tell you that he is going shopping. Your toddler is your shadow. He will do whatever you do and say whatever you say. Don't say or do anything you don't want him to repeat. Avoid profanity and such phrases as: "A nigger ain't shit," or, "Black folks never learn."

Little boys grow attached to their mothers at this stage and little girls to their fathers. When you have to go out, always explain where you are going. Never slip away or mislead your child. Tell him you are going to work, or to visit a friend, or shopping. Tell him in the simplest possible way.

Until they are about three years old, children fear abandonment, especially if you haven't always been with them. Don't ever tease your child that you are going to desert him. The fear that is aroused may be beyond quick repair.

By the time your child is two, he should have twenty teeth. Show him how to use a toothbrush. Don't compare his awkwardness with the skill of older children and make him resent brushing his teeth.

Discipline is of utmost importance for the two-year-old. Help him achieve what appears to be difficult for him, such as tying his shoes. Demonstrate by letting him put his hands on the string with you so that he can feel he is actually doing the job.

There are many things that he will be able to accomplish. There are also many things he will not be able to handle. Whatever you do, do not harass and push him. Allow him to develop at his own pace. Bear in mind that every child does not follow the same pattern. Allow for differences.

27

Your Child – Two Years to Four Years

A two-year-old is a sociable and friendly being who speaks to everybody in sight and gladly answers the telephone for you. He understands most of your conversation; enjoys being tidy; is independent and can feed and bathe himself, in a manner of speaking; and he likes to try to dress himself. Some children are toilet trained by the age of two with only an occasional accident. Nighttime training takes a little longer but may be accomplished before the third birthday.

If you have kept your infant clean, he will wish to be clean. If you have kept him happy, he will remain happy. If you have been too harsh with him, he will show harshness. If you have given him love, he will give love. If you have given him fear, he will show fear. If you have spent time teaching him, he will continue to want to learn. If you have been rude or loud with him, he will be rude and loud. If you have given discipline through praise, he will remain a well-disciplined child and will show it through his manners. In brief, the first two years of your child's life are very important to his total behavior.

Your two-year-old should be about twenty inches taller and

weigh about fourteen to twenty pounds more than he did at birth. It becomes evident now whether a child is left- or right-handed. The hair grows faster, with proper care. Don't braid it too tightly as this may cause a scalp infection. The feet may be a little flat, but there is no need for concern unless it causes problems.

Your child must have a yearly physical examination. The two-year-old should have completed all of his immunizations with the exception of his second polio and D.P.T. booster, which is due at the age of five. There is no need to test him for sickle cell anemia unless he has shown signs of the disease. His blood pressure should be tested, especially if there is a family history of hypertension.

If your child has begun to have difficulties digesting milk, he can get the nutrients contained in milk from cheese and many of the green and leafy vegetables. You should continue to give him vitamins daily.

Your child is now able to handle a lot of situations. He can put on his coat if you teach him how. One method is to place the coat flat on the floor, front opened, facing upward, and the top (hood) toward the child's body almost between his legs. Have the child stand with his legs parted. Now he must bend over to slip his hands into the sleeves. In this position, have him flip the coat over his head. The coat, including the hood if one is attached, will go on without any problem. He will enjoy this for two reasons: it's fun and he is learning to do something for himself.

He will make many attempts to put on his socks or tie his shoe-strings. He may not be able to accomplish this before he is three, but don't discourage him. Be gentle and patient with him and teach him how to handle these routine activities.

The two-year-old may show aggression if he is faced with a situation where he feels he must protect himself or his belongings. He may react by biting, holding on to the article, and screaming. All of this is normal. Don't become alarmed or angry. Tell him that he must learn to control his temper.

If he has older sisters and brothers, they will help him to learn

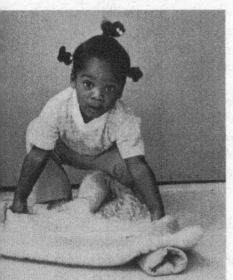

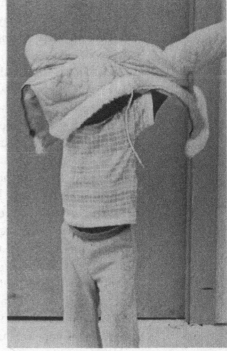

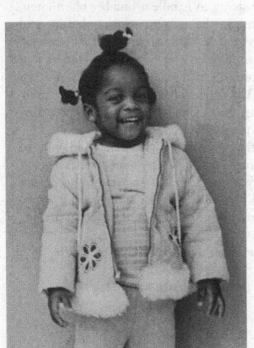

to live with other people. If he is an only child, you should provide playmates. If you are a working mother, and many black women are, place him in a day-care center or with a day mother who will not only keep him from hurting himself, but also provide for his other needs as well.

Julia was placed in a day mother's home because her mother worked. For ten children, all under five, Mrs. Smith, the day mother, used a very small, fully furnished room, about 12 x 15 feet, with eight additional children's rocking chairs and two playpens. She also had a small play area with a picnic table outside, but this could not be used during the winter months. The parents had to bring food.

Mrs. Smith liked children, but she was very impatient. When Julia originally started staying with her, she had a well-developed vocabulary, better, in fact, than the average two-year-old's. Her speech was clear and she was able to express herself fluently.

Severely limited in her ability to handle a number of children, Mrs. Smith had them sitting in their chairs most of the day and provided no learning activities. If one of the children became active, one could hear Mrs. Smith scream profanity throughout the neighborhood. She constantly told them to "shut up" if they talked or asked questions. And so Julia began to have speech problems. By the time she was three, her vocabulary had decreased and she could no longer express herself clearly.

You must check out the facilities where your child will be spending most of his waking hours. The environment has a great effect on your child's ability to grow up as a sociable being. It can also affect his appetite, and his ability to learn and achieve.

Wherever you take your child for day care, look for the following:

1. A variety of play activities and a fenced-in play area.
2. Children of his own age or close to his age.
3. Activities that will promote interest in other people.

4. An environment where he is not constantly confined or told not to do something.

5. A day mother or teacher with a warm personality.

6. A place where warm nutritional foods are served.

7. A rest area for each child.

8. A place where positive discipline—not beatings or other child abuse—is practiced.

9. An environment that fosters good speech and language habits.

10. A place where music, books, stories, puzzles, and dramatic play are available.

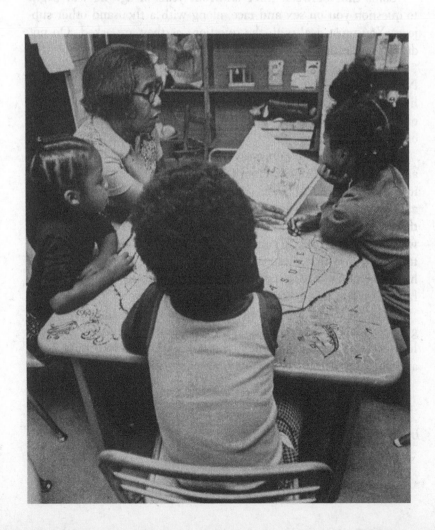

11. A reasonable number of adults to provide care.

If your center or day mother does not provide these essentials, consider another arrangement.

You may decide to take your child to a relative or friend instead. If you do so, speak with them about providing learning activities, as well as other children for him to play with.

The child between two and four years old is very observant and quick to pick up everything from you and others in his environment. It is extremely important that you and whoever the child spends most of his day with have the child's basic physical and mental needs in mind.

Some time between three and four years of age he will begin to question you on sex and race, along with a thousand other subjects. You must deal with the questions as they are asked. Do not dismiss a question with "Shut up" or "I'm busy."

Your discussions on sex should be accurate, brief, and casual. Normally you don't have to approach the child on these matters; he will ask, if you haven't already instilled fear in him. Don't giggle or become tense because of the subject. Never tell a child that sex or genitals are dirty.

Do not be negative in answer to questions about color. For example, you should not tell him that he is dark because blacks made it to God's stream of water just before it ran dry and were only able to get enough water to lighten the palms of their hands and the bottoms of their feet. Even though it is a comical, light-hearted way to discuss color, it suggests that being dark is an undesirable trait. Tell him that there is no need for him or anyone to defend his color. Once this is instilled into your child, he will be able to face the world in a positive manner.

Your child will be talking a lot at this age. At times you may get tired of hearing him talk. You must learn to communicate with him effectively. Not only must you talk with him, you must listen as well. This is the basis of a strong parent-child relationship.

Your child may also become partial to one or the other parent. While he will do almost anything his mother asks him, he may not listen to his father. Don't interfere with the less favored parent if he is trying to get the child to obey. Let the two of them work it out unless the situation becomes violent or uncontrollable. If this happens in your presence, simply take the child out of the heated environment until things cool down. Don't join in the temper flare by yelling at your partner or the child. Don't discuss the incident in the child's presence. This will only lead to more violence and may possibly cause long-lasting emotional stress for both the child and your mate.

28

Your Child –
Four Years
to Six Years

Between four and six your child grows quite a bit in mind and body. He loses his baby stomach as well as the last of his baby habits. He feels that he is capable of doing a lot of things now, and he is right. He is able to dress himself without too much help (shirts or blouses may go on backward, but don't worry). He is also able to handle his toilet needs without your help.

If you haven't been actively motivating your child to learn, do so now. He will soon be entering school, where the competition of life begins. Prepare him for this meeting. This means teaching your child how to live in an environment without you and still feel secure.

Most children stop taking naps during this period. It isn't necessary for them to nap if they are healthy. However, if you insist on your child's going to bed, he may just lie there and relax his body while using his mind.

You must now teach your child about privacy. Tell him not to enter your bedroom without knocking.

Your four-year-old may enjoy helping you set the table. Let him do so to make him feel that he is an active part of the family. His appetite may increase and he may accept a greater variety of foods. Even so, don't load his plate and then push him to eat it all. Give him small servings and allow him to ask for more. In this way, you will not have to nag your child about the "rising cost of food."

If you believe in having the entire family sit and eat together, you must have patience with children this age, especially five- and six-year-olds. They are active and may find it difficult to sit through a long meal. Begin teaching your child table manners, but don't order him throughout the meal to sit up straight, stop singing, and so on. Many parents are so concerned about the rules of etiquette that mealtimes become the worst part of the day for a child. If you make him nervous while he is eating, you may cause him unnecessary emotional and physical stress. Let him enjoy his meals and he will find them to be a time of family pleasure.

It should also be pleasant to linger and talk at the table after dinner. Allow your child to stay and listen if he wants. It is good for him to hear his parents discussing events of the day, family situations, or politics, or simply jesting.

Children this age are very active. Don't form a habit of referring to your child as "bad" if he is energetic. As long as he is controllable, behaves when you tell him to, and is not destructive, he is normal.

Avoid nagging your child. Many parents criticize their children all the time, making unrealistic demands upon them. "Johnnie, don't play in the dirt." "Rosa, your mouth runs like a bell clapper." "Janice, sit up straight." "Bernard, don't walk on the backs of your shoes." "Ella, don't put your elbows on the table." "Sam, you are going to be just like your no-good father." "Gloria, I am going to be on you like white on rice." This goes on day after day. Such talk causes tension, and children develop habits such as tongue sucking, nose picking, and nail biting. It may also contribute to hypertension, juvenile delinquency, and inferiority complexes. Talk to your child about things that annoy you and explain why, but don't nag him.

One of the things you must warn your child about is meeting strangers. Tell him that he must not ride in a car or talk to adults without your permission.

If your child is still bed wetting at this age, it is best to discuss the problem with him without embarrassing him. Ask him to think about what happens just before he wets the bed. Explain that normally he would have experienced a dream or nightmare. In most cases, the dreams entail situations where he believes he is using the toilet. Tell him that when he begins to dream he should immediately awaken himself and go to the bathroom. In the begin-

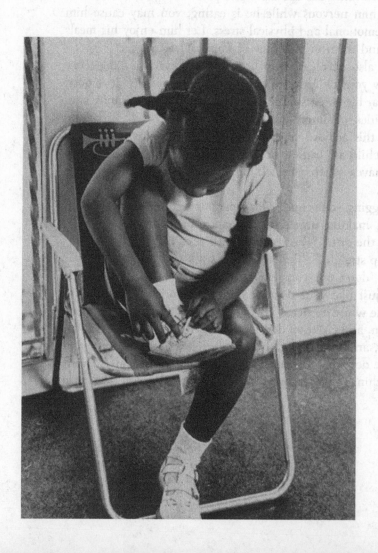

ning, he may not catch the first few drops, but once he makes the connection between the dream and the bed wetting, his bed-wetting problem will be over. If this does not work, take your child to see a doctor. He may be suffering from a medical problem, such as infection or a malformation of the urinary tract.

During this period your child will begin to lose his baby teeth. Explain to him what is taking place and assure him that it is a natural process. Many parents place a dime under the child's pillow during the night in exchange for the missing tooth. The gift is supposed to be from the "fairy godmother" or the "tooth fairy." If he asks who his fairy godmother is, show your child a picture of a black lady. This is especially necessary in a society like ours where he may learn to associate good acts with any race other than his own.

This is the period to give your child some systematic teaching about his blackness. Take him to see black and African art; tell him about black people in history and in today's life; read him black poetry, stories, and folk tales. Most children only know about a few black historical figures such as Dr. Martin Luther King, Jr., and Dr. Kwame Nkrumah. There are hundreds of blacks who have made significant contributions to the civilized world. Introduce your child to them.

Make sure that the books you find give the true facts. For example, some books assert that Hannibal was a white man. Hannibal was, of course, a Moslem Moor from North Africa respected by blacks for his role in the leadership of a group of African people.

Help your child develop a sense of responsibility. Teach him to respect his own property and that of others. Give him specific duties around the house such as putting his toys away after he has finished playing. Let him help you with the dishes. Send him to the store or next door with a message. If there are younger children around let him help change diapers or get the baby a bottle. Give him the opportunity to make decisions rather than always follow orders. It will help him to assume responsibility later in life.

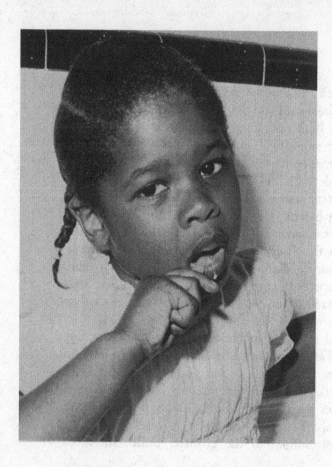

During this period your child should be able to use numbers, differentiate coins, recognize colors, and know the letters of the alphabet. He should also be able to tell his full name, address, and phone number. Of course, he can know these things only with your help and involvement.

A child this age has great imagination and may make up all kinds of stories. Don't accuse him of telling lies. Let him tell you his story and then say that it was a good "story" even though he may have wanted to make you believe it.

However, if your child has done something wrong and he fears punishment, he may just lie to you, a common reaction in this age group. To best overcome this avoid leading him into a lie. For example, say, "Dave, do you know where daddy's shoes are?" Not, "Dave, did you take daddy's shoes?" which could cause him to freeze up and deny everything, or put the blame on another member of the family. As you can see, the first approach is better, but only if spoken gently. There is a proverb, "Never call a dog with a whip in your hand." The same holds true for children.

If you and your mate are in constant disagreement, you are bound to affect your child's emotions. If you must argue, do so privately. An occasional disagreement is natural, but fighting is out. Control yourself—for your child's sake.

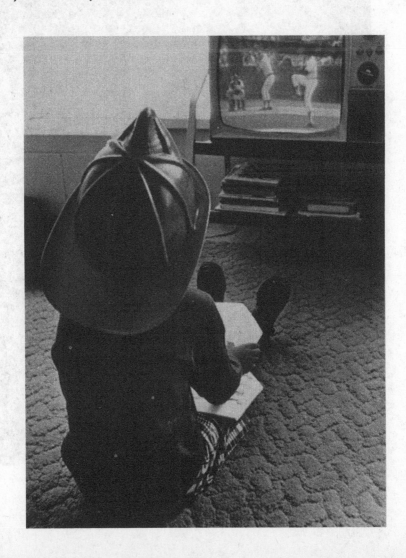

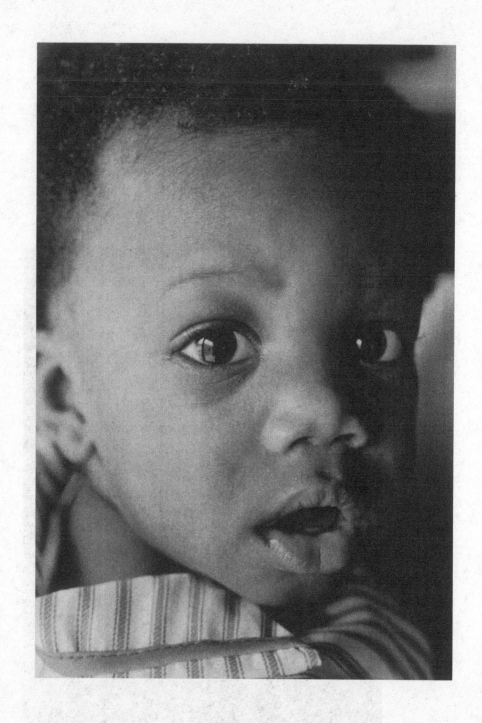

Part Three

Common Problems and Their Care

29

Accident Prevention
and First Aid

Accident Prevention

One of the first things you should do as new parents is accident-proof your house. This does not mean that you must place everything under lock and key. It does mean, however, that you must take precautionary measures to protect your child.

Your infant will be explorative. He will be curious. He will want to taste and feel things. Since most black infants reach this stage fairly early, you should begin now to look for hazardous things around your house. This will help keep down the number of accidents and also save you from having to say "no, no" too often.

You should check your house for hazards, and be sure to check for things that will cause fires or burn the child. You should place a guard across stairs and screens in front of fireplaces; keep cleaning materials in a special area; keep the floor clear of pins and needles; keep medicines locked out of reach; keep dry-cleaning bags packed away; put away sharp objects such as knives and scissors; guard against loose plaster and lead-painted objects; never leave lighted cigarettes in an ashtray; keep pot handles turned away from the front of the stove; keep electrical cords out of reach; and, most of all, keep an eye on your child.

CAR TRAVEL. You should always place your child in an infant

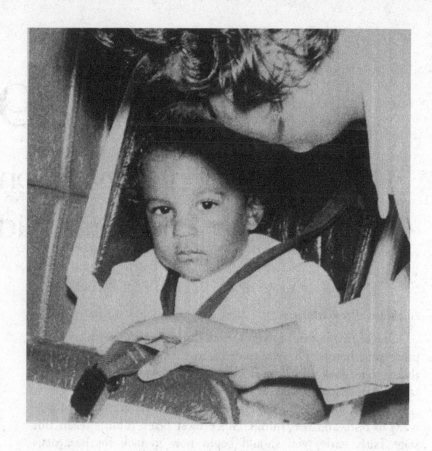

seat while you are driving and fasten it securely with a seat belt. Never allow your child to ride without a seat belt and never allow him to stand in the car while it is moving even if he is next to you or on the back seat.

First Aid

ARTIFICIAL RESPIRATION. If your child stops breathing as the result of an accident or because he is in shock, proceed with artificial respiration at once. The first moments are extremely important, so do not hesitate even long enough to call a doctor. Do not administer artificial respiration unless breathing has ceased. To administer artificial respiration you must:

1. Lay the infant on his back and remove any objects from his mouth and throat that you can reach without difficulty.

2. Put your hand under his neck to raise it, and tilt his head back by lifting his jaw.

3. Put your mouth over the infant's nose and mouth and breathe with a quick but mild force. (Babies breathe faster than adults.)

4. Remove your mouth while you inhale your next breath and breathe into the infant's mouth and nose again.

Check to see if the infant's chest moves up and down. Even if it does not contract after several tries, do not give up. Continue to perform artificial respiration until you get medical help.

FALLS. If your infant falls from a relatively high place he will no doubt cry for a few minutes and may suffer some swelling. Put a cold compress on the affected part. If he contines to cry for more than fifteen minutes, refuses to eat, vomits, shows signs of unusual sleepiness, pain in his head, or paleness (examine the palms of his hands), you should check with your doctor immediately.

FEVER. You can take a quick temperature reading of your child by feeling his forehead. But you must also keep a thermometer in your house for a truly reliable measurement. When a child is sick, the doctor's first question is: "Does he have a fever?" By this he means: Have you taken his temperature with a thermometer?

The normal body temperature is 98.6 degrees. This can vary anywhere between 98 and 99 degrees (measured with an oral thermometer). If your child's temperature should go too far below or above his usual range, get medical attention.

There are two types of thermometers for taking temperatures —oral and rectal. Before taking a reading, always shake the thermometer down to at least 95 degrees. It is not advisable to use an oral thermometer to take the temperature of a child under three years of age because of the danger of his biting it. Use a rectal thermometer.

This is how to do it. Hold the baby on your lap, with his face

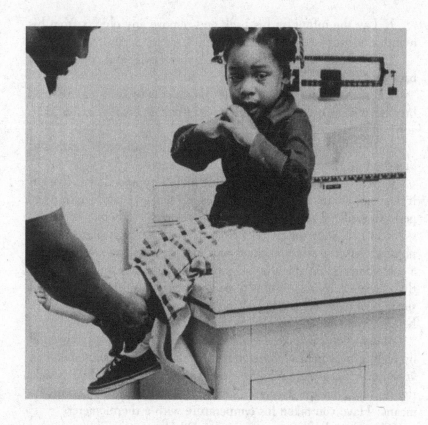

down. Apply petroleum jelly to the tip of the thermometer, spread the baby's buttocks, and insert the thermometer about an inch into his rectum. Let it stay there for at least two minutes. Be sure to hold the baby still. Holding his ankles usually restrains him. Rectal temperature readings are usually one degree higher than oral readings, so 99.6 degrees rectally is normal.

If it is not possible to use this method, you may take a baby's temperature under his arm. Hold the arm down for at least five minutes. A normal reading is usually between 98.6 and 99.6 degrees.

A child three years old or more can have his temperature taken orally. Slip the thermometer under his tongue for at least five minutes.

Clean the thermometer with alcohol after each use.

To read a thermometer, turn it so that you see where the mercury (the dark area) stops. Each line on the thermometer indicates a number. The long lines indicate the whole numbers, the smaller lines indicate fractions. For example, between 98 degrees and 100 degrees you will see one long line, which is 99 degrees. (Some thermometers also have a long line with an arrow for the normal reading of 98.6 degrees.) Between 99 and 100 you will see four short lines, which indicate 99.2, 99.4, 99.6, and 99.8 degrees. Most thermometers read in this manner up to 106 degrees.

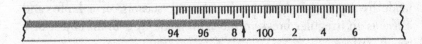

Thermometer Markings

Infants normally run higher temperatures than adults. However, if your child's temperature is above 100.4 degrees, you should take steps to bring it down. Here is what to do. Remove his clothes and wrap his body (not his head) in a towel dampened with water and alcohol. Pat him gently all over for a few minutes. Then dress him lightly, cover him with a receiving blanket, and let him rest. If his temperature remains high after this procedure has been repeated at least twice within a two-hour period, check with your doctor.

Some infants experience brief *convulsions* if their temperature gets too high. Should this happen, place your infant on his stomach and raise his chin so that he can breathe more easily. Clear his mouth of food and place a spoon or washcloth in his mouth to prevent him from swallowing, biting his tongue, or choking on his saliva. A doctor should be called immediately.

CHOKING. If your baby has swallowed an object and is choking, hold him upside down by his feet and slap him sharply several times on his back. Do not try to get the object out by prodding in his mouth because you may push it farther down. If you are unable to release the object from his throat, rush him to your nearest medical emergency center.

Should your baby stop breathing before you can reach the medical center, begin mouth-to-mouth artificial respiration (see page 154). Do not give artificial respiration to your child if he is still breathing.

WOUNDS. There are four basic types of wounds—abrasions, cuts, punctures, and tears. An *abrasion* is caused by rubbing or scraping off the skin. A *cut* is a straight slice through the skin made by the sharp edge of a knife, razor, or glass. A *puncture* is a deep wound made by a pointed object, such as a nail, scissors, or a knife, and a *tear* is an irregular break in the skin, made by a blunt object or a rough surface.

To treat a wound, be careful not to touch it with anything that is not clean. Wipe off as much dirt as possible with a sterile gauze or cotton, or hold the wound under running water. After this, apply a mild antiseptic to the area.

To control bleeding of the wound and to prevent infection, cover the area with a sterile gauze pad. Now apply a bandage over the pad, but not too tightly.

If the wound is deep and bleeding is profuse, do not try to clean it out; seek professional medical attention.

BLEEDING. You may be able to control bleeding by elevating the injured part of the body above heart level. After elevating the wound, apply a sterile gauze pad. If this is not adequate, pressure should be applied, holding a sterile cloth directly to the injury.

If bleeding does not cease, seek professional medical attention at once.

RAT BITES. Wash the area of the bite with soap and warm water. Then take your child to the nearest medical emergency center for further examination and treatment.

OTHER ANIMAL BITES. Wash the wound immediately with running water and soap to remove the saliva and blood. Apply a sterile gauze. Take the child to your nearest medical center or doctor. If possible, have the dog or other animal captured and delivered to the health department, so it can be checked for rabies.

BEE STINGS. Try to remove the stinger, then apply a paste of baking soda and water to the sting. Cover with a light bandage and keep moist. Some children may be very allergic to the stings of bees and wasps. If the reaction is severe, take your child to a doctor for treatment and consult him about treatment for any future stings.

SCORPION STINGS AND BLACK WIDOW SPIDER BITES. Almost immediately after the child has been bitten, he will experience very painful muscle cramps and abdominal pain. Before calling a doctor, give first aid: Tie a clean cloth tightly about two inches above the sting or bite if it occurs on the leg or arm, and keep in place for at least five minutes. It is not necessary to cut and suction the wound. If medical help is not immediately available, pack the bitten area in ice for two hours and hold this part of the body lower than the rest. Keep the child at a normal body temperature by covering him with a blanket if necessary.

BURNS AND SCALDS. If the burn is mild, apply a baking-soda paste or tannic-acid jelly. Cover with a sterile gauze. Make sure that the bandage is not on tightly.

If the area has blistered, be careful not to break the blister since infections can easily occur if this skin covering is removed.

Ice or cold water can also be used on burns and bruises.

Severe burns, of course, require immediate medical attention.

SPLINTERS. Apply a mild antiseptic and pick out the splinter with a sterilized needle or tweezers. Try to get the area to bleed a little, in an effort to wash out the wound. If possible, cover with a bandage or sterile dressing.

SHOCK. You will recognize shock if your child's face becomes pale, if he has a cold sweat, a rapid pulse, and irregular breathing, and is weak and nauseated. If these symptoms occur, keep him warm, with his body flat and his head low. If he is still conscious, give him a glass of something warm to drink. If he stops breathing, administer artificial respiration immediately. Rush him to the nearest emergency treatment center.

POISON TAKEN BY MOUTH. Quick action is extremely important if your child has swallowed a poisonous substance. Give first aid at once. Then call a doctor, hospital, or fire department to get help.

If your child is conscious, give him as much water or milk as he can drink, to dilute the poison. Other antidotes are: milk mixed with egg white; or milk mixed with flour, starch, or mashed potatoes to the consistency of a thin paste.

Induce vomiting if the substance swallowed is: after-shave lotion, camphor, arsenic, antifreeze, bichloride of mercury, boric acid, cologne, perfume, disinfectant, insect or rat poison, oil of wintergreen, rubbing or wood alcohol, ink, moth balls, hair dye, iodine, lead (found in paint), liniment, nail-polish remover, tobacco, zinc compounds, weed killer, poisonous plants, and contaminated food.

Also induce vomiting for aspirin, heart medicines, iron tablets, opium, codeine, paregoric, heroin, morphine, sleeping pills, headache and cold medicines, tranquilizers, birth-control pills, and diet pills containing barbiturates. The labels on many of these items will recommend specific antidotes.

To induce vomiting: Tickle the back of the child's throat with your finger; or give him at least one-half glass of warm water mixed with a tablespoon of salt or a teaspoon of dry mustard. Repeat, if necessary, until the stomach has been emptied. While the child is vomiting, lay him face down, with his head lower than his hips.

When vomiting has stopped, take the child to a doctor or hospital as soon as possible. If you do not know what poison he has swallowed, take a sample of the vomited material with you for laboratory tests. Keep the child's body warm by wrapping him with blankets, but do not allow him to become overheated.

Do not induce vomiting if the child is unconscious or in shock, is having convulsions, has burns around the mouth, or has swallowed furniture polish, gasoline, kerosene, cleaning fluid, ammonia, lighter fluid, lye, pine oil, turpentine, insect spray, drain cleaner, fire-extinguisher fluid, or a strong acid.

FOOD POISONING. Foods that have not been refrigerated properly, especially in hot weather, can develop the harmful bacteria that cause food poisoning. This is frequently true of food prepared with mayonnaise, such as potato salad, chicken salad, or sandwiches; or of food containing custard fillings. About two hours after the affected food has been eaten, the child may experience pain and cramps in the stomach, nausea, and vomiting. Induce vomiting if it does not occur naturally. Administer warm water after the vomiting has stopped, and keep the child's body warm.

Botulism is a severe form of food poisoning caused by bacteria sometimes found in improperly canned meats, fish, vegetables, and soups. It can be avoided if the canned food is boiled for 15 minutes before eating. The symptoms of botulism are nausea, vomiting, possibly diarrhea, and abdominal pain. After 12 to 24 hours, fatigue, blurred vision, difficulty in swallowing, and weakness are experienced. If you suspect that your child has eaten spoiled food, immediately follow the first-aid steps given above and then take him to the nearest medical facility.

PLANT POISONING. Only a small number of children are poisoned by eating plants, although there are many plants that are poisonous in whole or in part. These include many types of wild mushrooms and numerous house and garden plants, such as hyacinth, daffodil, elephant-ear, rosary pea, castor bean, dumb cane, mistletoe, autumn crocus, iris, star-of-Bethlehem, lily of the valley, bleeding-heart, rhubarb, rhododendron, azalea, jessamine, red sage, caladium, philodendron, burning bush, holly, poinsettia, sweet pea, and wisteria. Induce vomiting when poisonous plants are ingested.

It is best to instruct your child not to eat *any* plant leaves, flowers, or berries, unless you tell him it is safe.

In case of contact with plants that irritate the skin, such as poison ivy or poison sumac, wash the exposed area thoroughly with plenty of soap and water. Then wash with rubbing alcohol and rinse with clear water. If a severe rash develops and begins to spread or ooze, take your child to a doctor.

SKIN CONTAMINATION. Should your child's body be exposed to a poisonous or caustic chemical, immediately drench the skin with water, in the shower or under the hose, even while you are removing his clothing. Cleanse the skin thoroughly with lots of soap and water. If the chemical has burned the skin, treat as you would a burn from heat. Do not use a chemical antidote.

EYE CONTAMINATION. If a chemical substance or irritant has gotten into your child's eye, hold the eyelids apart while you flush the eye with water for not less than five minutes. Do not treat with a chemical antidote.

INHALED POISONS. The most common inhaled poisons are carbon monoxide, found in car exhaust, and cooking gas. Treat by carrying the child to fresh air immediately. Loosen all tight clothing. If he has stopped breathing, give him artificial respiration. Wrap him to keep his body temperature normal, and take him as quickly as possible to a doctor or hospital.

The best way to prevent poisoning is to instruct your child on substances that may be harmful to him and, most important of all, by keeping all potentially dangerous medicines and chemicals out of his reach.

30

Immunizations
for Infants
and Toddlers

A full-term baby at birth receives a fairly high degree of passive immunity from a healthy mother. These protective substances are further boosted in breast-fed babies by colostrum (which has an anti-infectious property) for the first few days after delivery. So, for the first few months of life the full-term baby who is kept clean and fed properly is relatively free of serious communicable diseases. But as the colostrum content decreases and the passive immunity disappears the baby must receive further immunization.

Vaccinations and immunizations are given at varying times during childhood to protect the child against communicable diseases, preventing a variety of complications which may cause permanent disability or even death.

The following is a discussion of these protective measures.

SMALLPOX. Primary smallpox, though no longer required in the United States, is given between fifteen to eighteen months of age. It is an injection of the antigenic agent, which, when effectively done, leaves a small scar at the site of inoculation. A few days after the injection has been administered, a small blister should appear. Sometimes pus is present and a fever may develop after the first week. Avoid giving the child a tub bath for the first four or five days since the blister must be kept dry. A bandage that can allow air to flow through should be used only if the child tends to scratch or pick at the scar. It is best, however, to keep the scar uncovered.

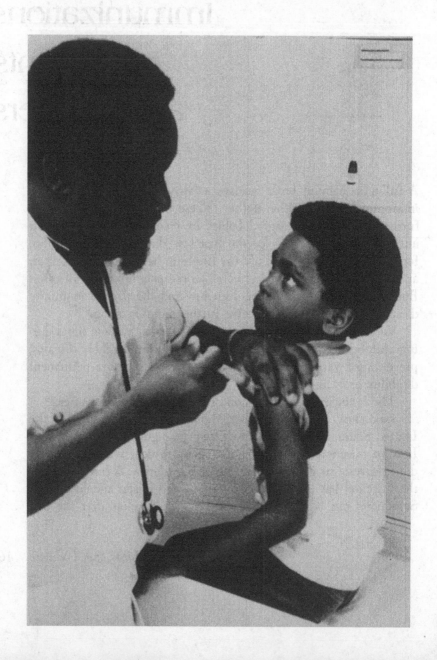

If the blister oozes, wipe it gently with a piece of cotton moistened with alcohol. The smallpox vaccination must be repeated every five years for adequate protection, but it is needed only for foreign travel in certain countries.

DIPHTHERIA, WHOOPING COUGH (PERTUSSIS), AND TETANUS (D.P.T.). These three inoculations constitute the basic immunization against diphtheria, whooping cough, and tetanus and can be given in combination at the same time. The first immunization is given at two months, the second immunization at four months, and the third at six months of age. The first booster is given at eighteen months, the second at five years, and a booster every ten years thereafter. A mild fever and tenderness and swelling around the injected area may occur after the inoculation. The baby may also become fussy. To minimize these side effects, your doctor may recommend one-third of a baby aspirin and warm compresses. The side effects should last only for a few hours and no more than two days.

POLIOMYELITIS. This disease is now much less widespread. Formerly associated with infants and called "infantile paralysis," it is now known to strike older children and adults as well. Caused by a virus found in the intestines, it affects certain nerves and leaves muscles supplied by these nerves partially or totally paralyzed. The vaccine should be administered by mouth at two, four, and six months of age. By providing your child with this protection, you are also contributing to community immunization. Normally, there is no reaction to this immunization. If one occurs, consult your doctor.

MEASLES, MUMPS, AND GERMAN MEASLES. The viruses of measles (rubeola), mumps (epidemic parotitis), and German measles (rubella), although different and causing different clinical diseases, when isolated and standardized can be combined into a single vaccine and given when a child is one year old. The prevention of measles is of great importance to infants and toddlers. The disease itself is not serious in a well-nourished child. There are, however, several potential complications among poorly nourished children, including upper respiratory and intestinal inflammation and, in rare cases, infections of the middle ear and sinuses. Some 0.1 per cent may develop inflammation of the brain and emotional disturbances. Mumps and German measles are not serious infections for the infant and toddler, but mumps can cause sterility in the male later in life, and German measles in pregnant women can damage the fetus, sometimes causing multiple severe malformations. Immunization for these diseases during infancy can provide permanent protection. In rare cases, fever and a light rash may occur as a reaction to the vaccine.

Here is the recommended program for these vaccinations and immunizations.

SMALLPOX

Before foreign travel, where required, or between fifteen to eighteen months of age and then, if necessary, every five years.

POLIOMYELITIS (three doses)

1. Two months of age
2. Four months of age
3. Six months of age
First booster—eighteen months of age
Second booster—five years of age

DIPHTHERIA, WHOOPING COUGH (PERTUSSIS), AND TETANUS (D.P.T.) (3 doses)

1. Two months of age
2. Four months of age
3. Six months of age
First booster—eighteen months of age
Second booster—five years of age
Every ten years thereafter

MEASLES, MUMPS, AND GERMAN MEASLES

Twelve months of age

Other Tests

Although tuberculosis (TB) is not considered among the communicable diseases of childhood, all children should be tested for the disease at one year of age and at regular intervals. Babies and young children can catch TB easily and should be kept away from people who have the disease or who have a cough of unknown origin.

Your doctor or clinic will give you are record of your child's inoculations. Keep it. This record will be needed when the child enters school, goes to camp, enters military service, or wants to travel abroad.

31

Infectious Diseases

The frequency and seriousness of communicable diseases among young children is related to inadequate diets during pregnancy and environmental factors after birth. These environmental factors include personal hygiene as well as home surroundings.

Many infectious diseases only strike children who are born with an inadequate amount of passive immunity, and they are prevalent among low-income families, where health education and living conditions are below average. Although a few viral infectious diseases are passed by the mother to the fetus, most of them could be avoided with proper diet and good hygiene.

Phyllis was the youngest of four children. Since her mother was their sole provider, she spent her days with a neighbor who kept eight other children, all under two. At fourteen months she had suffered no major sickness except for a cold or running nose periodically. One morning Phyllis's mother was awakened by her cry of anguish. She discovered the child had a temperature but took her to the neighbor's anyway. In the evening the child still had the temperature and had convulsions and vomited. Her neck was stiff and she was suffering chills. Phyllis was rushed to the hospital but died within six hours.

She had been fed with a plastic bottle throughout the day, continuously refilled with different liquids without being washed. She also slept with that bottle during the night. The family lived in a warm climate, and there were mosquitoes, roaches, and rats around. The doctor diagnosed her illness as bacterial meningitis and related it to an inadequate diet and poor hygiene.

Willie Mae had three children. She was unmarried and had a very low income, so she put them on a diet of ground-up table foods and skimmed milk before they reached six months of age. All of them suffered slow mental and physical development, frequent colds, and several types of infections. Willie Mae's children were always very clean and so was their home. Obviously they were affected by their poor diet.

Infectious diseases may be divided into four groups, based on the infecting agent. They are: viral, bacterial, and fungal infections, and parasitic infestations. Each is discussed below.

Viral Diseases

The organisms responsible for this group of diseases among infants and children are spread from person to person in a variety of ways such as coughing, sneezing, spitting, and contact with excreta (bowel waste), skin, and mucous membrane of a diseased person. Spreading of the germ is aided by unhygienic and unsanitary practices.

In situations of overcrowding, poor personal hygiene, and poor environmental sanitation, cases of viral infections are more likely to exist, particularly in the young child. Certain vitamins, minerals, and protein elements in the diet of infants and children are known to promote resistance to some of these viral diseases. These nutritional elements also help the victims of the disease to recover.

The most common viral infections among infants and children are:

COMMON COLD. Usually not very serious. Normally starts with

a dry, stinging feeling in the nose and within twenty-four hours develops into running nose and eyes, sneezing, coughing, and difficult breathing. Some children experience fever, muscle pain, weakness, and sweating. If fever is present for more than two days, see a doctor, since your baby may be suffering from the flu. Treatment: baby aspirin, fruit juices, and plenty of rest.

INFLUENZA (FLU). High temperature, chills, runny nose, coughing, muscle soreness, and headaches are normally the signs of influenza. The symptoms are usually more severe than those of a common cold. Treatment: baby aspirin, fruit juices, and plenty of rest. Highly contagious. Contact your doctor if temperature lasts for more than two days.

MEASLES (RUBEOLA). Vaccine is now available (see page 163). The first symptoms are fever and cough with runny eyes and nose. About three days later, small bluish-white spots appear in the mouth. The rash later breaks out on the body. Measles is highly contagious during the period of fever and runny nose. The child should be kept away from other children who have not had the disease. Calamine lotion is good to stop the itching. Aspirin may be given for fever. See a doctor.

GERMAN MEASLES (RUBELLA). Immunization is now available (see page 163). The first sign is usually a reddish rash. The glands behind the ears and back of the head swell. The child may also develop a sore throat and have a mild rise in temperature. This disease is highly contagious and lasts about three days. It is very dangerous to pregnant women, as it may affect the unborn child. Treatment consists of baby aspirin and plenty of fluids and bed rest. Consult a doctor.

MUMPS. Immunization is now available. Child normally develops fever with pain and swelling around either one or both jaws. Swelling is sometimes noticeable under the chin. The disease is very contagious, and particularly dangerous to a male adult since it may cause sterility. Keep the child isolated until swelling is gone. Pain may be relieved with hot or cold applications. Baby aspirin should be taken for fever. Avoid tart foods such as orange and grapefruit juices as they may cause a burning sensation in the mouth. May last from a week to ten days. Consult a doctor.

CHICKEN POX. Symptoms begin with headache, slight temperature, and small patches of bumps that develop into blisters in the center. The blisters will discharge and dry into scabs. This disease is highly contagious before and after blisters appear. May last a week to ten days. Child must be kept in isolation and the pocks (blisters) must be kept clean by washing with soap and water. Do not allow the child to scratch blisters. Keep fingernails cut low since scratching may cause permanent scars on the body. Itching can be relieved by rubbing blisters with calamine lotion or a paste of baking soda and water. Consult a doctor.

INFANTILE PARALYSIS (POLIOMYELITIS). Immunization is available (see page 165). Fever, drowsiness, headache, vomiting, stiffness in neck and back, and pain in limbs are normally the first symptoms. Paralysis may appear from one to four days after first symptoms. This disease is very contagious during the first week. The child must be taken to the hospital.

FEVER BLISTERS OR COLD SORES (HERPES SIMPLEX). Child usually has high fever and is very restless. Chills are sometimes present. The skin lesions are blisterlike and may appear in large numbers on the body, face, mouth, or gums, sometimes overnight, and they continue to appear for three to seven days. This disease is contagious. See a doctor.

VIRAL WARTS. There are several types of warts which vary according to location on the body and the child's age. Common warts usually occur as dry, oval, gray growths on the hands. Juvenile warts are small and flat, and usually occur on the face. Filiform warts are threadlike and are found on the eyelids and neck. Digitate warts are found on the face and scalp. Genital warts are normally found on the penis or around the vagina.

Warts spread by direct or indirect contact, through barber shops, swimming pools, restrooms, and other public places. New lesions may occur if they are accidentally made to bleed. Most are present only on the first layer of tissues even though some do involve deeper tissues. See your doctor.

ECZEMA. Patches of irritated itching areas on the skin. Many shapes and sizes. If scratched, wetness occurs and scabs appear. Usually shows on the cheeks, around the navel, under the diaper, or around the leg of the diaper. Sometimes appears behind the ears, in the groin, on the abdomen, or on the back of the legs. Rash in diaper area is usually dry and thick. *Caution:* A child with eczema should not be vaccinated and should not be around people who have been recently vaccinated for smallpox. Keep him away from wool, including clothing and floor coverings. See your doctor.

MOLLUSCUM CONTAGIOSUM. This is a common viral disease which occurs in young children. It is manifested by small white pearly bumps that can spread to other areas of the body through scratching. These lesions usually appear on the face and are often on the eyelids themselves. See your doctor.

Bacterial Diseases

With breast-feeding, a nutritional diet, and good personal hygiene and home sanitation, bacterial diseases affect young children less often than viral diseases. Also, preventive inoculations are available to fight against the common bacterial diseases of diphtheria, whooping cough, and tetanus.

Other common bacterial infections include:

SCARLET FEVER. Begins with headache, fever, sore throat, and vomiting. The pulse rate is rapid. Reddish rash normally follows twenty-four to seventy-two hours later. May cause kidney disease. Treatment is available (penicillin). Consult your doctor.

PNEUMONIA. Upper-respiratory-tract infection. Symptoms include stuffy nose, fretfulness, and low appetite during the first days followed by a sudden high fever, restlessness, and difficulty breathing. Consult your doctor immediately.

STREP THROAT (BACTERIAL SORE THROAT). Difficulty in swallowing is normally the first symptom. Check for enlarged tonsils. Give recommended dosage of baby aspirin and fruit juices, and see that your child gets plenty of rest. A mouthwash can also be used for the older child. If fever occurs or if soreness lasts for more than twenty-four hours, consult a doctor. An untreated sore throat that is caused by the Streptococcal bacteria can lead to rheumatic fever and kidney disease.

SAND SORES (IMPETIGO). Most common in warm climates. Begins with pimples or blisters on the face or legs which quickly become cloudy and rupture. Blisters have a yellowish crust. This infection is highly contagious, and medication is needed for cleaning and anointing infected areas. Bed linen and clothing of the infected child should be changed and sterilized daily. Take him to a skin specialist.

HAIR SORES (TRACTION). A common problem in the young black female between two and ten years of age is this recurring bacterial infection on the temple areas of the scalp. One reason for this condition is the increased traction put on the hair as the result of tight braiding, a popular way to keep hair well-groomed and manageable. Some hair styles (for example, corn row) have been known to cause keloids in African women. Many older girls and adult females suffer this problem because they roll their hair too tightly. The first signs of this condition are small red pimples around the roots of the hair that become white with pus. The infection also causes hair loss. Treatment consists of an antibiotic rubbed into the infected area, as well as medication taken by mouth. It is best to use preventive measures. Do not braid or roll hair too tightly. Hair should be kept loose.

FOLLICULITIS. Redness of the scalp with pus formation and itching. Hair loss is also a symptom. It is contagious. Consult a doctor.

Fungal Diseases

Fungal diseases among infants and children are relatively few. These are essentially associated with prematurity, poor nourishment, poor personal hygiene, and unsanitary surroundings.

Common ailments in this group are:

THRUSH. Initial symptoms include sore mouth, poor appetite, and a whitish covering of the tongue and oral cavity. Consult a doctor.

RINGWORM OF THE SCALP (TINEA CAPITIS). Scaly patches on the head with broken or lost hair. It is contagious. Consult a doctor.

TINEA VERSICOLOR. More frequent in warm climates. Light-colored spots, patches, or large confluent areas on the neck, trunk (chest or back), face, or portions of the arms or legs. In infants, normally found on the face and diaper area. Scales when scratched. Use a mild antifungal ointment, and consult a doctor.

RINGWORM. A fungus infection of the skin, hair, or nails. It is contagious and should be treated. The spot usually itches and heals from the center, forming the rings. See a doctor.

Many fungal skin lesions in children are generally not serious, but they frequently cause emotional trauma in parents who think that the lesions may cause permanent physical damage.

Parasitic Infestations

These infestations, seen from time to time in young children, are usually associated with poor families. Barring rare complications, they are not a threat to life.

The most frequent infestations are:

LICE. There are two species of lice that produce infestation of the scalp, body, and pubic area. The most common in children appear in the hair and scalp, and often on the eyelids as well. It is a long-lasting condition. The lice feed on blood and leave small reddish spots, followed with pus and itching. On the scalp, itching is normally the first noticeable symptom. Consult a doctor for proper medication and care.

SCABIES (IMPREGNATED MITE). They appear chiefly on the face, between the fingers, and around the groin. Itching begins about a month after infection. Welts form—whitish, threadlike, zigzag—which open into small oozing areas when scratched. This is a contagious and chronic infection. Consult your doctor.

PINWORM. Pinworm infestation can be very bothersome and persistent. The symptoms are an itching and burning sensation in the rectum, loss of appetite and weight, and sleeplessness. The worms are sometimes seen in the child's stool or in his bed clothing. Take him to see a doctor and also practice good personal hygiene and home sanitation. The doctor should examine the entire family, since it is generally a family disease even though the initial focus is on the symptomatic child. The treatment generally involves all of those who have close contact with the bedding and clothing of the infected child.

HOOKWORM. This condition is most often found in the South and warm weather countries. The worms penetrate the skin, and work their way to the lung, following a complicated course through the body. Hookworm is often found in children who do not wear shoes. It causes diarrhea, restlessness, and loss of weight. This condition can cause intestinal blockage. Consult your doctor.

32

Environmental, Genetic, and Medical Problems Common to Blacks

There are many hereditary and environmental factors that affect the newborn infant. These factors determine his emotional stability, his physical strength and health, the shape of his body, the color of his skin, eyes, hair, and a variety of other things. About 2 per cent of the world's population has some defective genes. The resulting condition varies from extremely harmful to almost negligible. Genetic counseling is helpful in avoiding serious genetic problems.

The percentage of black infants born with serious congenital or birth defects is relatively low. Most of the serious health problems in the black population are caused by environmental factors and can therefore be avoided, particularly if you and your mate practice good health care before conception.

Environmental Problems

LEAD POISONING. This disease predominantly affects the young poor and black. The effects of lead are exerted on the central nervous system (brain and spinal cord), causing mental retardation and poor coordination. The major sources of lead poisoning are paint and plaster containing lead; furniture, especially cribs, painted with lead paint; fruit covered with lead pesticide; and lead toys.

It is now illegal to use lead paint in the United States, but the majority of blacks live in buildings that still have multiple coats of old paint and plaster. Small children are the victims of lead poisoning not only because of sociological factors but also because they sometimes have a condition called "pica." Pica is the craving to eat certain things. Many small children put everything into their mouths, but pica goes beyond this. Some believe that these children like the sweet taste of lead paint, and others say that an iron-deficient diet causes them to crave paint.

The symptoms of mild lead poisoning are headaches, weakness, loss of appetite, vomiting, irritability, and abdominal pain. Severe poisoning manifests itself as anemia, hypertension, convulsions, and lack of coordination. It is important for inner-city mothers to watch for these symptoms so that if lead poisoning occurs it can be diagnosed by a physician and treated promptly.

SUDDEN INFANT DEATH SYNDROME (CRIB DEATH). "SIDS" is usually diagnosed when an infant is placed in his crib in seemingly good health and is found dead, without apparent reason, several hours later. Statistics show that SIDS occurs more often among black male infants of low birth weight and in families of low socioeconomic status. Most of the deaths occur in infants between two and three months of age and during cold weather, when upper-respiratory illnesses are common.

To date, no one has been able to determine any specific causes of the disease. The signs that have been found in most SIDS victims are an inflamed respiratory tract, water-swollen lungs, and hemorrhages on the surfaces of certain vital organs. Infants sometimes show signs of having "struggled for breath" before dying. SIDS is not hereditary and has not to date been associated with neglect by parents.

Many researchers feel that SIDS victims might have suffered a chronic respiratory ailment before death that had gone undetected. Therefore, have your child checked for respiratory-tract infections after birth and specifically during the critical periods mentioned.

STUTTERING. Stuttering usually relates to environmental and psychosocial problems. It is often related to a child's emotional state. Parents who are anxious for their child to succeed are likely to correct his grammar or pronunciation all the time. The child then becomes nervous and begins to stutter. The condition is more common in male children and begins between two and five years of age.

It can be eliminated with proper guidance and parental help. If your child begins to stutter, give him your complete attention when he talks, without interference or pressure. If the condition grows worse or is not corrected in later childhood, take him to a speech and hearing specialist.

Genetic and Medical Problems

KELOID. A keloid usually follows injury to the skin caused by a sharp object. It is a scarlike lesion that keeps growing and enlarging.

Keloids occur predominantly in black people. The lesions vary in size and shape. The most common locations are the face, arms, legs, and chest. Perhaps one of the most distressing locations is the ear lobe. This occurs in young girls after their ears have been pierced. If a child has had a history of keloid formation, ear piercing should not be done without consulting a physician. The removal of keloids is sometimes an unsatisfactory treatment because they often recur.

Currently X-ray therapy, injection of the keloid with hormones, and surgical removal are employed.

MONGOLIAN SPOTS (LIVER SPOTS OR BLUE MARKS) are dark

blue lesions, stemming from a lower layer of the skin, that make the skin opaque. All races have this blue layer in their skin makeup. When manifested, the lesions are usually found as bluish spots on the buttocks or lower back, although they may be present anywhere. The condition is common in black and oriental babies. The size of the spots varies from very small to patches covering the buttocks and lower back. With time they decrease in size, and they disappear before the child is five. No treatment is necessary.

MILK SPOTS (VITILIGO). Vitiligo is an acquired disorder in which the substances that give color to the skin disappear. The condition is seldom found more than once in the same family.

It can occur at any age and on any part of the body. However, most frequently it appears in the areas around the eyes, face, mouth, anus and genitals, and on the fingers, backs of hands, and tops of feet.

Vitiligo occurs also in people without color, but it is more psychologically damaging to blacks because it is more apparent. As a result, treatment for the condition also includes psychological counseling.

Dr. John Kenny of the Howard University Vitiligo Clinic has done more research on the disorder than anyone and has come up with several effective methods of treatment. The most common involves painting the affected area with a medication called Psoralen. After one hour the area is exposed to a black light. This creates an artificial sunburn which leads to the gradual appearance of the natural color.

This medication is also administered in pill form. The patient must then wait for two hours before being exposed to the black light. Although black light is used, the best light is actually natural sunlight.

In severe cases of vitiligo, where over fifty per cent of the body has lost its color, some physicians use a compound that will remove the color from the rest of the body rather than restore color. Much consideration should be exercised before undergoing this treatment because the loss of color—in effect, changing from black to white—inflicts severe psychological damage on many people.

Also, many physicians are against this method, since color acts as a protection for the skin, and once the color is bleached out, the skin becomes more susceptible to damage by sunlight and to the subsequent development of skin cancer.

You should know that some chemicals used in heavy cleaning agents may also cause loss of color in the same manner as vitiligo. People working as maids or janitors in industries that use these strong chemicals are the most common victims of this condition. Before using a strong cleaning agent, check its content to make sure it does not contain tertiary butylphenols. Treatment for this disorder is the same as that for vitiligo.

LACTASE DEFICIENCY. Lactase is the substance in the body that breaks down the sugar lactose, which is found in milk. It has been shown that deficiency of lactase is more common in the black population. When milk is ingested, people who have lactase deficiency can experience bloating, abdominal pain, and diarrhea. Most of the adult black population is unable to drink large quantities of milk.

Research done by Dr. Norman Kretchmer and Dr. Frederick Simmons of the National Institute of Child Health revealed that an adult's inability to drink large quantities of milk is normal. They concluded, in fact, that the ability of mammals (including humans) to drink milk without complications after the nursing period is abnormal. If your child is unable to drink milk, he can get the nutrients supplied by milk from other sources, including any aged cheese, such as sharp cheddar, where lactose is almost nonexistent.

GLUCOSE-6-PHOSPHATE DEHYDROGENASE DEFICIENCY. This disease is seen frequently in black males. It is also seen in a small percentage of black females. Italians, Greeks, and other Mediterranean, Middle Eastern, African, and oriental ethnic groups, as well as Sephardic Jews, also suffer this deficiency. The disease is more severe in whites than in blacks. The susceptible person may become anemic about 58 to 96 hours after he has ingested or come into contact with such substances as aspirin, mothballs, and some antibiotics and antimalarial drugs. The patient usually recovers, although jaundice and hemoglobin in the urine may be present in severe cases. (Jaundice is a yellowish discoloration of the skin and the white part of the eyes caused by anemia or liver disease. Hemoglobin is the protein matter in the red blood cells.)

UMBILICAL HERNIA. Umbilical hernia is common among blacks. It is due to an imperfect closeness or weakness of the muscle covering the abdomen. Thus, instead of the navel being flat, it is pushed out by the abdomen in a pouchlike fashion. There is no cause for alarm because umbilical hernia rarely presents any real problem. Many of the measures taken by well-meaning people such as applying a navel band, taping a quarter over the hernia, and rubbing vitamin E oil on it are useless, and often irritate the skin. Even the largest umbilical hernias usually close without treatment by the time a child is five years old. It should be noted that an inguinal hernia, which occurs in the groin or area of the sexual organs, is more serious and should be evaluated immediately by a physician.

TIED TONGUE. Many black parents are concerned when the tongue of their newborn infant is connected at the very tip with a threadlike piece of flesh to the floor of the mouth. One should only be concerned with this condition if it prevents the child from speaking clearly. Most children with this condition do not suffer a speech defect, and the tongue should be left alone. Surgery is seldom necessary.

EXTRA FINGERS AND TOES. A number of black infants are born with six fingers or six toes. Most require no medical attention since it is merely a cosmetic problem. If the parents desire to have the extra finger or toe removed, they should discuss it with their doctor during the child's infancy.

MULTIPLE BIRTHS. Twins and triplets are more common in

black families, and 30 per cent of the twins are identical, formed from one fertilized egg. Naturally, the feeding and clothing of two or three infants can place an unexpected economic burden on a black family. With the use of fertility drugs, an increasing number of families outside of the black population have given birth to twins, triplets, or quadruplets.

HIGH BLOOD PRESSURE (HYPERTENSION). This is the most serious health problem in the black community. Susceptibility is hereditary, and the condition is accelerated with stress. It has recently been found in young children. Most doctors neglect to test the blood pressure in children because they consider hypertension an exclusively adult problem and because the blood-pressure level for young children has not yet been established. Even though hypertension is usually not as severe in the young, you should insist that your child be given a blood-pressure test, especially if there is a history of hypertension in your family.

SICKLE CELL ANEMIA. The vast majority of people with sickle cell anemia are black. However, sickle cell disease has been reported among nonblacks in Europe, India, and the Middle East. We now know that sickle cell anemia originated biologically as a protective mechanism against malaria. Even today, malaria remains a problem in some parts of Africa. People with sickle cell anemia are more resistant to certain forms of malaria. This is Nature's way of protecting the African people.

As we have already explained on page 62, there is a significant difference between sickle cell *trait* and sickle cell *disease*. A person with sickle cell *trait* does not have the disease and needs no treatment—a very important fact to understand, because this harmless condition occurs in one out of every ten American blacks. On the other hand, the *disease* occurs only once in every five hundred American blacks.

How does sickle cell anemia affect a child? The most common complaints are decreased appetite, weakness, fatigue, and pain. The pain is usually in the arms, legs, back, and abdomen. The eyes may also turn yellow and the child may become pale (check the palms of his hands).

In an infant, the disease may not show itself until after the baby has suffered an infection normally involving his lungs or intestinal tract. He may exhibit high temperature, paleness in the skin and palms of hands, irritability, poor eating, and enlarged heart, liver, or spleen. He may also suffer swelling of the hands and feet.

In a child between two and four years of age, swelling of the hands and feet may be the first indication of sickness.

When the symptoms of the disease become pronounced, the patient is said to be having a crisis. He should be taken immediately to the doctor for treatment.

Sickle cell anemia cannot be cured, but modern methods of treatment have considerably brightened the outlook for the patient.

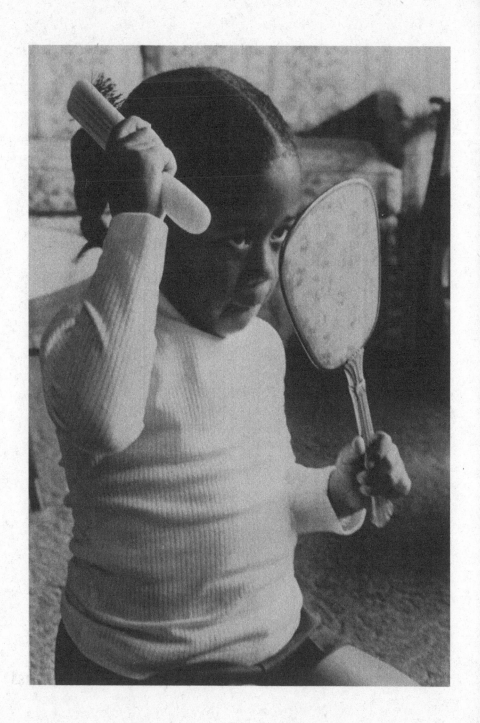

Part Four

Educating the
Young Child

33

Discipline

Discipline is essential in developing self-confidence and self-respect. Children need discipline to grow and feel secure. It is discipline that makes the need for punishment unnecessary. Discipline allows each individual to adjust his conduct to an acceptable social standard.

Discipline begins at birth. When your baby is hungry, he learns to wait until you have prepared and brought him his food; he learns that he cannot receive his food instantly. If you acknowledge his needs and please him, he will be content. When he grows older, he will want to please you in turn. Discipline breeds love and respect.

Before a person can show love and respect, he must form a conscious personal relationship. For the infant, this relationship begins with his parents. He draws on it later in his conduct with individuals not related to him. Your child learns to live with other people through the discipline you share with him. Teach him the advantages of good manners. Only through discipline can he learn to cope with the demands of his environment.

Your child will learn discipline and acquire a sense of values from the examples you set for him. You cannot tell a child, "Do as

I tell you to, not as I do." If you use profanity, or show disrespect to your partner in marriage, your child will follow your example. If you place greater value on drinking or smoking pot than on eating wholesome foods, your child will do the same. On the other hand, if you teach him to respect you and other members of the family, show respect for him, praise his achievement, and guide and comfort him through new experiences, you are on the right track.

As a parent, you must maintain authority with your child. Indecisiveness breeds confusion. A positive attitude breeds respect. This does not mean that you must be distant with your child and not show love and affection. It means that you must set up reasonable standards as a guide for him to follow. It means that you must also live by those standards. When a child has guidelines to follow and examples to imitate, he will understand just how far he can go. For example, if you do not wish your child to put his feet on the sofa, you must tell him so. You must also let him know what the penalty is for putting his feet on the sofa. If he chooses to disobey, he knows what the consequences will be. If you do not make him pay the penalty, you will lose your position of authority; he will lose his respect for you. You will show him that you (1) are not a person of your word and cannot be trusted; (2) may possibly fear following through with the penalties; and (3) are indecisive.

If you sometimes pretend that you did not see your child disobey, you may undermine your authority. A child can sense that you are watching him, and will continually test you to see how far he can go. Be consistent in disciplining your child if you wish to remain in control. Once you have lost control, you have also lost your child.

You must learn how to criticize your child's behavior, not the child himself. Many parents are unable to do this. Yet it's easy to love a child and not like what he has done. When you tell your child, "You get on my nerves," you are telling him not only that he has done something annoying, but also that he, as an individual, bothers you. A child can accept the fact that you have rejected an act but he cannot accept being rejected as a person.

Many parents resent certain looks, habits, or attitudes in children simply because they remind them of someone they dislike or something their parents disliked in them. You must guard against such resentment because it will lead to needless conflict.

Some children need more discipline than others. Watch your child to determine his individual needs.

If punishment is due, restrict his activities or spank him. But

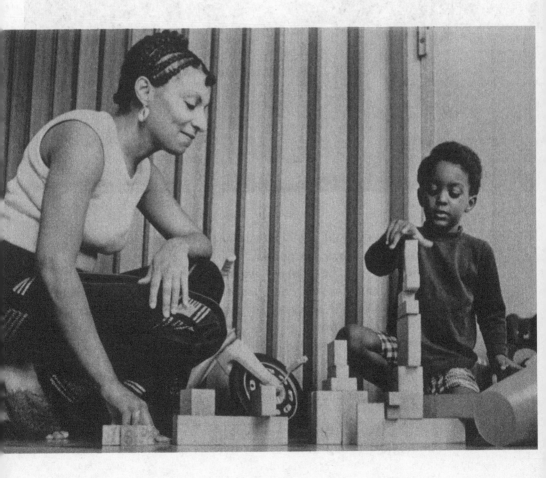

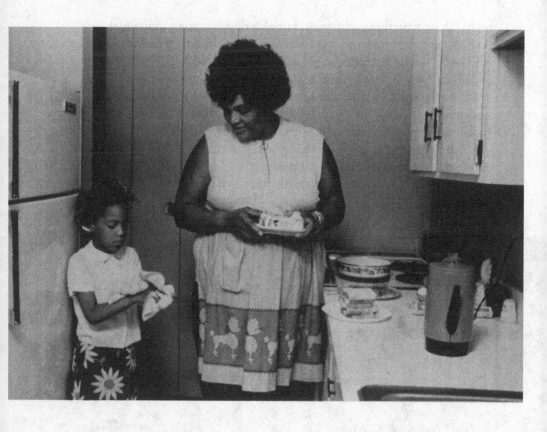

never beat your child. To beat is to instill fear or to defeat. This is not your goal when you punish.

Discipline can be achieved without physical punishment. If you set up limits for your child, and are consistent in maintaining them, it will not be necessary to punish. If he does not respect your limits, he is ready to pay the penalty. Never threaten a penalty you can't follow through with. For example, do not say, "Boy, if you break that glass I will bust your head wide open." Can he believe you? Although most black children sense what you mean when you make such a statement, you should still set up realistic penalties. Make the punishment fit the crime. Perhaps breaking the glass was an accident. Does this deserve punishment? If it was done intentionally, then you know your child is testing you, and he should be reprimanded. All children test, just as they all explore.

Teach your child to be a positive thinker. If your daughter should experience difficulties later in school or with her peers, do not say, "Poor Brenda. She is having a hard time." If you show pity, Brenda will develop self-pity and will never be able to rise above her own low opinion of herself. You must encourage her. She will get strength from your belief in her.

Do not allow your child to use blackness as an excuse for copping out. For example, many children find it easier to say that a poor grade was received in school because of his color than spend the necessary time studying or completing a required assignment.

The most effective form of discipline is praise. Your child will be more than happy to follow your desires if you praise him. Praise is also a tool for motivation. Before you can effectively praise your child, you must recognize his limitations or capabilities, you must know how far to push him to help him grow. If you overtax his abilities, both of you will be disappointed when he fails.

Your infant will begin to explore as soon as he is independent enough to move about. This is one of his major ways of learning. So allow him independence, within reason. Do not spend your whole day saying "no, no" to him. He will think that everything is a "no, no," and he will fall into that avoidable "terrible two's" category. A child will not go through this stage if he has been properly disciplined. "Terrible two's" stems from "terrible training." If he does something that endangers his health or seriously displeases you, try to explain it to him. For example, if he begins to explore the broken pieces of a plaster wall in your house, simply say to him, *"Plaster* is *bad* for you!'" He will be able to detect from the sound of your voice and the look on your face that he should not touch it. Needless to say, parents have the responsibility for removing such a danger. You must be consistent if you expect to succeed. If you ignore his playing with the plaster one day, and the next day he is able to eat some before you can stop him, you have allowed him to endanger his health.

You should not punish your child because he does something that annoys you. A child cannot understand punishment if he is unable to relate it to a specific wrongdoing. This is true for infants and children, and for adults as well.

Discipline also means teaching your child the advantages of good manners. This simply means being pleasant to other people.

Loss of parental control often leads to the battered child syndrome. Most parents guilty of child abuse are also victims of child abuse. If their parents undressed them, tied them to the bedpost, and beat them, they in turn will tend to punish their offspring in a similar manner. Sometimes they act impulsively. Victims of even small amounts of abuse as children may manifest its effect in later life, not necessarily with children, but with others they love.

Rodney remembers vividly the day his parents hung him by his feet over an opened outdoor toilet because he had told a lie. When he got married, he told his wife that she must live above suspicion. Whenever he thinks she has told a lie, he brutally beats her. Rodney always regrets beating his wife, but he continues to do so because of his prior conditioning.

Parents who are child abusers usually regret the pain they inflict upon their children. However, if they themselves were abused as children, their tolerance for tension is usually low. Tension is relieved when they strike out. If you recognize that you are a potential child abuser, if you discover that your child-abusing impulse is out of your control, you must seek professional help immediately.

Discipline is taught not only by parents. A child is in contact with many other people, such as his grandparents, babysitters, and teachers. You must tell them what your standards are. Most grandparents are more permissive with their grandchildren than they were with their children. If your child's grandparents are overpermissive, and you are unable to handle them, limit your child's stay with them. Your child will achieve more and appreciate more in a well-disciplined (not strict) environment.

You may want your child to have religious education, which can be very helpful to him in our complex society. His introduction to religion should not be difficult, boring, or frightening. On the contrary, it should be pleasant and enlightening.

Raising a black child in a world where color receives so much emphasis is indeed difficult. It requires you, as a black parent, to be especially competent in teaching your child to cope with the society while working for change. The system makes it difficult for a black child to have a good image of himself. Do not help to perpetuate the color-inferiority fallacy. Help him to become self-confident and self-satisfied.

When you say to your son, "You will never amount to anything," you are encouraging him to realize your prediction—become a delinquent, drug addict, or nothing. When you say to your daughter, "I am going to send you to college so that you can make it in life because you have the ability," you are giving her the necessary courage to achieve. It is almost customary in the black community for the daughter to be encouraged to achieve and for the son to work and struggle on his own. Children of both sexes need your encouragement and guidance. Please give it to them equally.

34

Sex Education

Probably the most serious handicap for many parents trying to teach their children about sex is their own misunderstanding of the subject. Many adults understand sex only in terms of sexual intercourse. Before you can encourage a healthy sexual attitude in your child, you must understand sex in all of its aspects.

Sex education begins when your child is born. When you hold him tenderly and he responds, he is developing sex attitudes. He is learning to appreciate love, tenderness, and physical contact.

Soon, he will begin to explore his own body. When you see him holding his genitals, be cool. Don't stop him or say, "No, don't touch!" Each child explores his genitals in the normal course of development. If it really bothers you to see him touching his genitals, remove the hand and redirect his attention to some equally interesting activity.

To educate your child on sex, you need not be stern and businesslike. It's not necessary for you to sit down with him and begin a discussion at a particular time. Sex education should be taught on a day-to-day basis, naturally, on his level of understanding.

A young child begins to learn about sex when he notices that his parents' bodies are shaped differently. He learns about sex as you teach him language symbols: man, woman, boy, girl. Even if he is an only child and has not seen the sex organs of other children or adults, he will eventually ask about the difference between man and woman, boy and girl.

When you teach your child the parts of his body, point out his genitals as well as his eyes, nose, ears, stomach, legs. Always explain the parts of the body to your child in correct terms. That paves the way for a natural and relaxed discussion of the more complicated aspects of sex in later childhood and adolescent life.

When your child asks questions about sex, and all do, you must give him true, direct answers. If you refuse, ignore him, or show tension, he may turn to someone else for this information and get the wrong answer.

"Where do babies come from?" is often the first question that parents find hard to answer. Be direct. If your child is asking about human beings, don't try to explain in terms of the birds and the bees. He will not be able to relate them to human sexuality. When he asks you why Linda and Lewis are different, first find out specifically what he wants to know. He may not have sex in mind. If he really wants to know why Linda is a girl and Lewis is a boy say to him, "Linda is a girl because she has a vagina. Lewis is a boy because he has a penis." If he wants to know more, explain that Linda has a uterus, where a baby will someday grow, making her a mother. If a boy wants to know about his ability to have a baby, tell him that he enables his wife to become a mother by planting a seed inside her body that will grow into a baby, making him a father.

In crowded apartments or houses, where children of different sexes must sleep in the same room and bathe together, curiosity about sex differences is evident much earlier. Children begin to play doctor and nurse and other sex games that require both sexes to participate. They also explore each other's bodies and compare sex organs—sometimes openly, on the front porch, sometimes in private under the bed. If you see them, do not frighten them or spank them. Say something like: "Oh, you want to see what Alex has, and he wants to learn about your body. You have a vagina and Alex has a penis. When you get older I'll explain more so that you can understand why your bodies are different."

Even if your children don't see you and your mate in sexual intercourse, they may hear your love sounds. Those children who have been exposed accidentally to the sex act itself may try to imitate what they have seen or imagined with one of their friends—opposite sex or like sex; it is usually not that important to them. A natural desire to imitate adult behavior is the real reason for mother-father, doctor-nurse, or boyfriend-girlfriend games, not sexual stimulation. Most children's sexual play is sparked by something they have seen, something that adults have tried to hide from them. Teach your children early not to enter your bedroom before knocking and receiving a response.

Should you see your young child imitating love-making, don't scream at him or spank him. Diverting his attention toward another activity will be sufficient. Normally, a child loses interest in sexual play once he begins school and his interests are expanded.

If you encourage conversation with your child, he will ask questions about sex without fear. If you are able to answer him without anxiety, the conversation should flow easily.

If your child doesn't ask questions, you may help him by reading books specifically designed to tell children about sex. At your public library you will find books such as *The Wonderful Story of How You Were Born* by Sidonie M. Gruenberg. Mrs. Gruenberg, a grandmother, has written a beautiful story for children up to age ten. The story is simple and the illustrations show people of all races involved in the natural phenomenon of having children. There are books for every age level. Check with your local librarian.

It's not a good practice to expose your child to sex books and magazines showing nude men and women. Young children cannot understand adult-oriented material, and adolescents may only be embarrassed or confused by such literature.

Children's naturally sensuous movements, such as swinging the hips, should not be magnified by your attention. Nor should they be teased about behavior predominantly associated with members of the opposite sex—a boy playing with dolls or wanting to wear mama's shoes.

Sex education also involves your relationship with other people. You must be exceptionally careful not to downgrade an absent mother or father. If you are a single parent, do not expose your child to a variety of lovers. It is fine to have friends, but until you have made a definite commitment to a love relationship, refrain from intimate gestures and love-making around your children.

The best sex education you can give your child is through the example you set for him as parents. If you love each other, show respect and affection for each other, and demonstrate responsibility, your child stands a good chance of growing up sexually healthy.

35

Learning to
Communicate

Much of our waking time is spent in communication with others. The fact that we can communicate (speak, write, listen, and read) through language is one of the most significant abilities which separates us from other animals. Because man has language symbols, he can pass on his culture, review his past, evaluate the present, and prepare for his future.

The average black child usually begins crawling and babbling around four to six months of age. These are his first steps toward independence and communication. Respond to your baby's sounds by talking with him in the language you wish him to learn, not baby talk. Your infant will try to imitate your speech. Express delight with his babbles. This will encourage him to learn. If you do not respond to his babbling, he may greatly reduce the use of his new-found ability.

How often have you heard a black parent say to his child: "Will you please shut up before you talk me to death," or "Don't bother me," or "You don't have to know why. Just do as I say." These parents are obviously not encouraging effective language development in their children.

Language development is related to the child's environment as well as his age. Talk with your infant by pointing out objects and people in his surroundings, as well as in books and newspapers and on television. Give him the opportunity to see at first hand what he has learned about in pictures. Allow him to see animals, fire trucks, soldiers, and nurses. When you take your child for a walk, say to him, "Mama and Edward are holding hands. We are walking to the store." In that one sentence he will probably pick up *mama, hands, walking,* and *store.* When you reach home you should say, "We are now at home. This is the apartment building

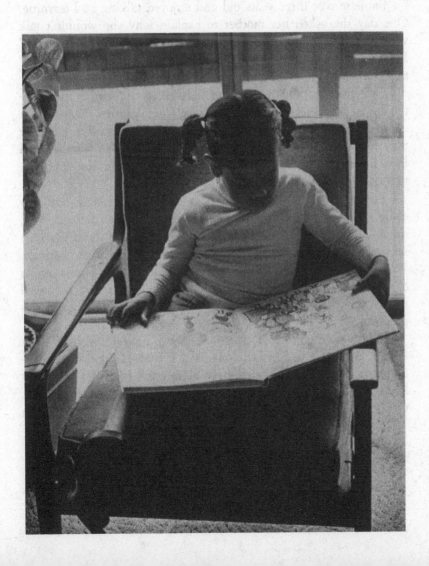

where we live." *Home* and *apartment* are now a part of his vocabulary. Even though he may not be able to express all of these six words, they are keyed into his mind for use in the near future.

When you dress your child, name the articles of clothing. Allow him to look at himself in the mirror. Refer to yourself as *mommy* or *daddy*. Point out his sisters or brothers. These practices will enable the infant to know himself and to label the objects or people in his surroundings. Children love learning to use words. If you fail to help or encourage this pleasure now, they may experience problems in learning later in life.

Paulette was three years old and enjoyed talking and learning. One day she asked her mother to explain why she wouldn't talk with her. Her mother replied, "I do talk with you, Paulette." Paulette answered, "No, mama, you don't. You only say 'Un huh' and 'Un un.' "

Paulette's inability to get her mother to respond in full sentences is not uncommon in the black community. Many such children are reluctant to express themselves verbally. Basically they fear being ignored or repulsed. Many are also handicapped by a limited vocabulary. Limited vocabularies are a result of limited conversations and limited exposure.

Too much television in the household routine may not only cause children to speak poorly but disrupt family unity as well, since families who spend their waking hours before the TV screen seldom talk to each other—except for requests to change channels.

Some children may seek verbal attention with a high number of questions. Your child's question approach to you may very well be his way of forcing you to talk with him and to recognize his presence.

When your child asks questions, never respond with "I don't know." Always give brief explanations. If a child asks you a question that you are unable to answer, simply tell him that you don't know but that you will look it up and let him know. And be sure to find out. When he says, "I saw the blue sky," you should not

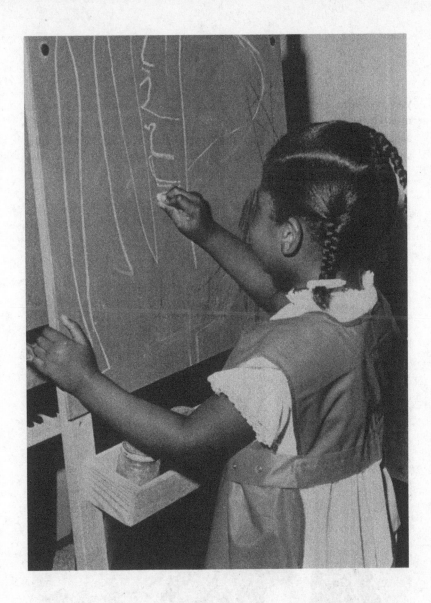

respond with "You did," without further recognition. Encourage the child by saying, "Really? Was the sun out, or was the sky filled with clouds?" With this approach, you communicate with your child and stimulate him to observe and analyze, to think.

Encouraging your child to communicate does *not* mean that

you must be an expert in languages. It does *not* mean that you must buy a lot of teaching aids and overwhelm your child with alphabets and numbers. It does *not* mean that you must make him spend a certain number of hours each day reading a book. It *does*

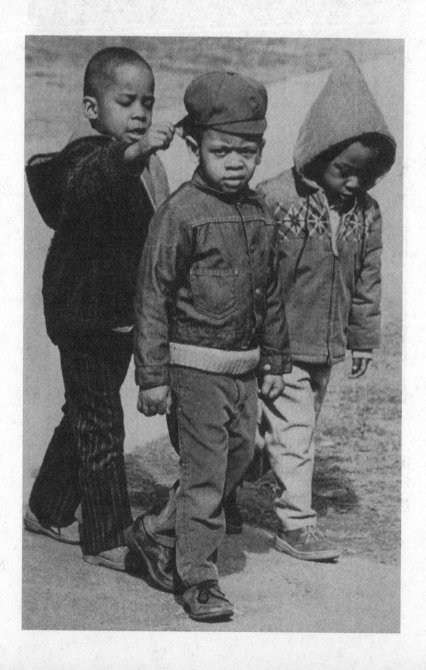

mean that you must spend time with your child. It does mean that you must show affection. It does mean that the two of you must be able to understand mutual language symbols, whether they be English, French, Greek, or Swahili.

Speech Disorders

It's not uncommon for young children to have speech and language problems. The first six years are the major years for a child's speech and language development. Any abnormality becomes evident during this period. If you suspect that your child is having speech and language difficulties, take him to a speech clinic or a doctor before the condition becomes serious.

Many parents are so anxious for their child to speak correctly they fail to realize that he must first go through a development process. They spend hours correcting his pronunciation or grammar. This type of pressure makes the child timid. He refuses to talk and often develops a speech disorder.

Standard English and Black English or Dialect

You must encourage your child to use the language that will enable him to communicate effectively in a given situation. Does this mean that you must encourage your child to learn language patterns outside his immediate environment? Yes, it does, especially in the United States, where the average black child eventually studies or works outside the black residential community. Only a lion understands a lion, and only a person taught a dialect understands that dialect.

It's your duty as a parent to explain the necessities of life to your child. Effective communication is a necessity of life, and the child must be taught the benefits of learning the language of his dominant society. If he moves to Spain, he must learn Spanish. This does not mean that he must disregard completely his own cultural language. It only means that he is providing himself with the tools to communicate effectively in his *dominant* environment.

All children learn to speak the language of their *immediate* environment. In countries such as the United States, parts of Africa, and the West Indies, a child must learn one language for his immediate environment and another for his dominant environment. By immediate environment, we mean the house and neighborhood—inhabited by parents, relatives, and friends—of the child's day-to-day life. By dominant environment, we mean schools, shops, and outside society in general. For example, in the United States a child from the black ghetto may speak a dialect of English in his immediate environment. However, when he begins school, he is *required* to learn standard English, the language of the dominant environment.

In a society where most books and newspapers are written in standard English, the child should learn to communicate effectively in standard English. In the West Indies, for example, the common spoken dialect is not the same as the common written language. This is also true in many other countries.

It is not difficult for a child to learn to speak and understand more than one language. The difficulty arises when people in his environment make disparaging remarks about his bilingual ability. This type of ridicule is the reason for such sayings as: "A tiger will not make fun of another tiger's stripes, but an elephant without a trunk will say that trunks are useless."

Karlene spent the summer in the North and soon picked up the speech patterns of the people around her. The day she returned to her Southern town a friend asked if she had talked with a mutual friend. Karlene replied, "I haven't seen him yet." Her friend laughed because Karlene didn't reply with the more familiar: "I ain't saw him yet."

Difficulty also arises when a black child starts school. If his parents have taught him to speak standard English he will be ridiculed by the other black children. If the child only speaks the language of his environment the teacher will show displeasure.

To avoid these situations, some black children learn early to communicate in both forms of English.

As a parent you must teach your child the importance of effective communication. Effective communication means that he must be able to speak, write, read, and understand the appropriate language of his dominant environment. Your child's ability to succeed depends upon his ability to communicate effectively in that environment. This is true today, it was true yesterday, and it will be true tomorrow.

36

Black Pride—
Let's Work Together

As black parents in a white-oriented world, there are specific steps you must take in order to establish a sound relationship with your child and thereby promote a sense of self-esteem in him. When we say self-esteem, we mean a child's growing up to love and respect himself and consequently able to love and respect others, particularly other blacks.

First you must realistically review your own ideas and experiences as a black person. Your clear understanding and acknowledgment of yourself as a black has a direct bearing on your child and how you relate to him. The first question is: Do you love yourself as a black person?

Most of you will say right away: "Of course I love myself." But have you ever wished your hair was straighter or your skin lighter? You may say no to that, but have you ever subconsciously felt inferior when you were in the presence of white or lighter-complexioned people? Do you think a baby who is born dark is not attractive? Have you ever felt envy toward a person with long, straight hair? Do you refer to hair as "good" or "bad" hair? Do you feel superior to other blacks when you have close white friends or when in the company of whites or people of other races? Do you subconsciously enjoy or dislike someone's company because of his complexion or race? Do you feel that a doctor is more knowledgeable, more competent because he is white? Do you claim that you go to the white lawyer because "he plays golf with the judge and can get you over?" Do you find it easier to accept the advice of whites? Are you more comfortable in a situation where you are the only black? When you see other blacks in your predominantly white school or neighborhood, do you wonder with disgust what they are doing there? Do you avoid speaking to other blacks because you are both black? Do you spend a lot of money on clothes because you feel clothes make you superior? Do you laugh at very dark people because of color alone? Do you make disparaging remarks about fellow black people because of their features? And are you guilty of looking at a newborn baby's fingertips or ears to see how dark the child will eventually be?

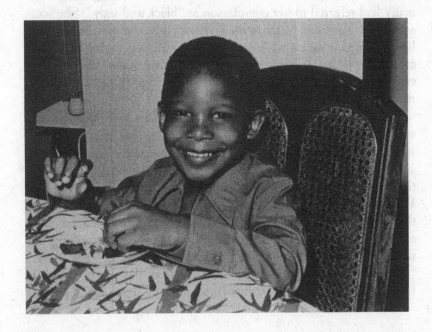

These are just a few things that we as black people do to promote the fallacy that only white is right. Although many of the attitudes described above may not be a part of you as an individual, they are still a very strong part of the black community.

No matter how often we say we are ready for the revolution—"Black Power"—as long as these things creep subconsciously into our minds or our actions, we are prolonging our slave mentality and most likely passing it on to our children. This is why the myth of black inferiority seems imperishable.

The ability to dig out and expose the roots of black inferiority lies within us. Forget who the first teachers of black inferiority were. That is no longer important. We are now the teachers, and the strength of our people depends upon us and how we handle our children.

Mary Frances was a very dark girl with small facial features and shapely body. No one had ever told her she was ugly although many had referred to her complexion as "black and ugly." She soon associated blackness with ugliness since only the girls who were light-skinned were called "cute." One day she was taking her usual crosstown walk to her grandmother's house when an old lady stopped her and told her she was very pretty. She thought it strange that the lady would make such a comment.

Shortly afterward, a man stopped her and also told her she was very pretty. As she continued her journey to her grandmother's, some young children playing on the sidewalk said, "Hi, lady, you sure are pretty!" With this, Mary Frances became depressed. By the time she reached her grandmother's she had broken into tears. When her grandmother asked her why she was crying, she told her that people had picked on her all the way there. When asked to explain what she meant, the teenager said, "They kept telling me that I am pretty and I can't be pretty because I'm too black."

Even though this incident occurred before the slogan "black is beautiful," the concept is still in the minds of many black people.

It is there because we are indirectly taught that black is ugly and, therefore, we are ugly, because our own people constantly make a mockery of themselves. They say things like, "Did you see how black he was, and those liver lips!" A man once told his friend that he thought the young lady sitting across from him was very pretty. His friend replied, "I can't tell, she is too black for me to see." Blacks also make comments such as, "Her hair is (snapping their fingers) that short," or, "His hair grows like watermelons in a patch—every knot stands out."

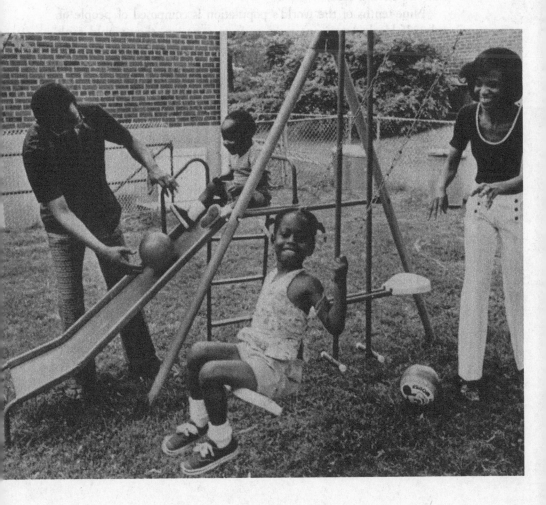

Adding to their disparagement of themselves they do just the opposite for white or very light complexioned people, or people with straight hair. Though many are trying hard to accept black as beautiful, deep within, the complex is there, even within families where the color range is wide. Sisters and brothers call each other black, yellow, or nappy head.

You must sincerely begin to rid yourself of the need to laugh at very dark people or call hard-to-manage hair "bad hair." Stop giving people of other races as examples of what we should do and how we should look.

Nine-tenths of the world's population is composed of people of color. If black Americans were to form a nation, they would rank number twenty-six in size among the more than two hundred nations and colonies of the world. The first civilized nation of the world was black. The first people of the world lived on the African continent. Why do we think we have to explain or defend blackness?

Virginia had a high-school teacher she tried to avoid because he always greeted her with the statement, "You sure would be pretty if you weren't so black."

Mamie returned home from school with scratches on her face. When her mother asked what had happened, she explained that she had been in a fight with a white girl. "Why did you fight her?" her mother asked. "Because she called me black," Mamie replied. "Would she have fought you if you had called her white?" "No," Mamie said, "it's okay to be white."

The need to explain or defend blackness perpetuates racial inferiority. Only when we as blacks cease to have that need can we live as a proud people. The roots of racism are deep. They have had a long time to grow. They have been well fertilized. They have been nurtured by many people, including some blacks.

Your child may not be able to recognize color differences among people until he is three or four years old. When he does, he will probably ask you about color. How will you explain color differences to him?

Tell your child that there are four basic color groupings—black, red, yellow, and white. He is a part of the black group, which originated in Africa. There are many shades of black.

You may tell your child that his color stems from a chemical in his body called "melanin." All people have melanin, but he has more, and that makes his skin beautifully darker.

Teach him to be proud of his blackness.

Index

Index

CPSIA information can be obtained
at www.ICGtesting.com
Printed in the USA
LVHW030230170520
655839LV00013B/531